Preventing Substance Abuse

Interventions that Work

Preventing Substance Abuse

Interventions that Work

Michael J. Stoil
Prevention, Intervention, Treatment Coalition for Health
Cincinnati, Ohio

and

Gary Hill
Conwal Incorporated
McLean, Virginia

Plenum Press • New York and London

WITHDRAWN

Library of Congress Cataloging-in-Publication Data

On file

ISBN 0-306-45454-8 (Hardbound)
ISBN 0-306-45455-6 (Paperback)

© 1996 Plenum Press, New York
A Division of Plenum Publishing Corporation
233 Spring Street, New York, N. Y. 10013

10 9 8 7 6 5 4 3 2 1

Printed in the United States of America

Foreword

Most experts in the field of preventive care acknowledge that much progress has been made over the past 15 years in the development, implementation, and promotion of strategies to reduce the health, safety, and welfare problems related to abuse of alcohol, tobacco, and drugs. While it is commonly agreed that "an ounce of prevention is worth a pound of cure," too often advocates for prevention struggle to name more than one or two examples that convincingly make this point. Researchers, planners, and practitioners need to know how successful prevention efforts have been thus far and what kinds of approaches have been most effective in various situations.

This book seeks to assist the field in this regard by discussing various substance abuse prevention strategies and programming. Its goals are to provide a conceptual framework for analyzing the progress that has been achieved in this field and to foster awareness and understanding of successful approaches to the problems of alcohol and drug use.

Preventing Substance Abuse does not intend to be conclusive or to offer the definitive answers to the prevention field. Research and applied experience in this field are still far from complete. Nor is it the intention of this book to infer that the approaches cited are the only ones worthy of consideration. Instead, by focusing on lessons learned and on promising practices from the past two decades, this book is dedicated to furthering the mission of encouraging the advancement of knowledge in the prevention of alcohol and drug abuse and related problems.

Jacqueline P. Butler, President
Prevention, Intervention, and Treatment
Coalition for Health (PITCH)

Preface

Preventing Substance Abuse is designed to help behavioral health practitioners, managed healthcare administrators, and community leaders sort through potential choices on drug abuse prevention. To meet this purpose, the book describes specific solutions that have documented evidence through rigorous evaluations that they produce desired change. Most of *Preventing Substance Abuse* takes the form of an informal guide to successful prevention programs, identifying their origin, implementation, outcomes, and—where possible—a current contact who can provide additional information and assistance. The two final chapters of the book are somewhat different: they address, respectively, general "dos" and "don'ts" of prevention, including knowledge gained from rigorous evaluations of programs that didn't work.

The authors and the national nonprofit Prevention, Intervention, and Treatment Coalition for Health (PITCH) believe that communities need straightforward analyses of what appears to work in reducing alcohol abuse and drug use. As managed care organizations and local jurisdictions assume more of the community prevention responsibilities that formerly were held by the U.S. Public Health Service, this need will continue to grow.

Preventing Substance Abuse meets this need by presenting "substance abuse" as a constellation of problems that cannot be resolved through a single set of prevention solutions. Its origin lies in the National Structured Evaluation of Alcohol and Drug Abuse Prevention, a project funded by the Center for Substance Abuse Prevention (CSAP) within the Department of Health and Human Services. Its focus on what has been documented from outcomes in the field rather than on theoretical perspectives of what *should* work is possible only because of the National Structured Evaluation's unprecedented review of successful prevention.

Acknowledgments

Assistance and guidance from many people contributed to the development of this book. The authors recognize the value of this early support, including the opportunity to review hundreds of unpublished documents describing the implementation and outcomes of prevention demonstrations funded by CSAP from 1987 through 1993. In particular, the authors acknowledge the support and encouragement of Michael Dana, Melvin Segal, Eric Goplerud, Gail Held, Kent Augustson, Mary Jansen, and Elaine Johnson, director of CSAP.

This work benefited from the dedication, expertise, and insights of a Technical Advisory Panel composed of five individuals with extensive experience in the evaluation of substance abuse prevention activities: Jacqueline Butler, James Emshoff, Roy Gabriel, William Hansen, and Eric Schaps. Their insightful critiques, and additional suggestions offered by John Swisher, shaped our approach to presenting prevention efforts that document effective performance through a methodologically rigorous evaluation.

We also acknowledge our debt to our colleagues at Conwal. Valued contributors to the earlier CSAP-funded project include John Sheridan, Paul Brounstein, June Bray, Charles Lupton, Carol Woodside, Kelly Hancock, Gayle Fenster, Brian Berkopec, and Danyal Ahmed. Michael Ney, Maryann Kramer, and Suzin Mayerson also provided invaluable assistance to the National Structured Evaluation while at Aspen Systems.

Alexandra "Nicki" Walters and Kim Kerson have been pillars of support during both the National Structured Evaluation and the preparation of *Preventing Substance Abuse*, organizing the records for over 1600 prevention projects and maintaining contact with the more successful efforts over several years. Kami McClelland and Ashley Ney spent hours searching for misplaced semicolons, run-on sentences, and more serious glitches in this manuscript.

Finally, we appreciate the support provided by Conwal's President, Everett Alvarez, Jr., and Executive Vice President, Kevin C. Riley, who made this effort possible.

Contents

5. Problem: Preparing the Ground for Prevention in Early Adolescence **55**

6. Problem: Preventing Drug Use in Secondary School 71

7. Problem: Intervening with Teenagers at Highest Risk for Addiction **89**

A Problem–Solution Approach to Substance Abuse

Former Surgeon General C. Everett Koop wrote in 1995 that the most important gains in prolonging life have come not from miracles of diagnosis and treatment in the late 20th century, but from the community prevention successes in the late 19th and early 20th century:

> [D]iseases are of two types: those we develop inadvertently and those we bring upon ourselves by failure to practice preventive measures. Preventable illness makes up approximately 70% of the burden of illness and associated costs. (Koop, 1995, p. 760)

In the same article, Dr. Koop noted that 35% of the causes of death today can be attributed to personal decisions to use tobacco, alcohol, or other drugs, or to maintain unhealthy patterns of activity and diet.

Future gains in wellness—and reduction of medical costs—depend on supporting personal decisions to enhance health. As communities have led prevention against infectious disease through vaccination and safer water and food, they must invest in prevention against "life-style" health risks.

This book is designed to help sort through choices on substance abuse prevention, including preventing abuse of alcohol and prescription medications. The premise is that decision makers benefit most from learning directly about successful attempts to reduce the rate of substance abuse rather than from generalized theories about what *should* work. To meet this purpose, this book describes specific solutions that have shown evidence through evaluations that they produce measurable change. Most of *Preventing Substance Abuse: Interventions That Work* takes the form of an informal guide to successful prevention programs.

The two final chapters of the book are somewhat different. They address, respectively, general "dos" and "don'ts" of prevention. The chapter on "dos" lists principles of implementation, funding, and decision-making. The chapter on "don'ts" uses knowledge gained from what has been tried and found to be unsuccessful to identify pitfalls that communities can avoid.

SUBSTANCE ABUSE: A CONSTELLATION OF PROBLEMS

All of the following situations can be defined as "substance abuse":

- A curious 10-year-old raiding the household liquor cabinet for a first taste of dad's bourbon
- An addict committing petty crimes to pay for heroin
- A young woman who doesn't stop smoking when she realizes that she may be pregnant
- A middle-aged rock fan who still likes to smoke marijuana when listening to Woodstock-era music
- A usually abstinent senior citizen driving erratically after consuming champagne at a wedding and painkilling prescription medication for sciatica
- A self-employed laborer spending a large chunk of the week's earnings on a weekend binge of alcohol and cocaine

The common thread among these situations is that they all involve use of alcohol or other drugs that poses risks for individual users and potential costs to society. Otherwise, they are very dissimilar behaviors. Their causes and cures differ, and the methods to prevent them differ.

Most drug abuse problems can be concisely defined by answering three questions:

- What drug is used?
- Who is using the drug?
- Under what circumstances is someone using the drug?

For some drugs, only the first question is necessary. All heroin use is substance abuse, for example, because the drug is very addictive, dangerous to physical and mental health, and illegal. For other drugs, all three questions must be answered. The opiate fentanyl, for example, has legitimate medical uses and is generally accessible only to clinicians. Abuse usually occurs when doctors or nurses apply fentanyl to nonmedical situations.

Table 1.1 defines several substance abuse problems in terms of users and situations. It intentionally makes no reference to ethnic or economic distinctions among users and only one reference to gender. One reason for these omissions

Table 1.1. Varieties of Drug-Related Problems Discussed in *Preventing Substance Abuse: Interventions that Work*

Type of problem	Drug used	Drug user	Situations in which used
Drug-affected babies (Chapter 2)	All drugs, tobacco, and alcohol	Women of childbearing age	During and/or after pregnancy
Family transmission of drug abuse (Chapter 3)	Illegal drugs	Adult(s) or older adolescent(s)	Recurring use while in contact with younger family members
"Gateway" drug use (Chapters 4–5)	Alcohol and/or tobacco	Younger than 13 years old	Any use other than religious
Adolescent substance abuse (Chapters 6–7)	Drugs and alcohol	Youth aged 13 to 18	Any illegal use
Drug addiction/repeat use (Chapters 7–8)	All addictive drugs	Usually older than 13	Chronic use of illegal drugs or alcohol
Adult substance abuse problems (Chapters 8–9)	Drugs and alcohol	Older than 18 to 21	Any use that risks adverse consequences

is that drug use patterns refuse to remain neatly defined by demography. For example, cocaine was widely distributed during the early 20th century, became identified with African-American users during the middle of the century, enjoyed resurgent popularity among high-income users during the 1970s, and returned as a drug of choice among ethnic minorities in the 1990s (for example, Casement, 1987). With few exceptions, defining drug users by education, income, housing status, or ethnic origin reinforces prejudices and hampers efforts to provide prevention to all in need.

HOW COMMUNITIES RESPOND

Communities differ on what they are willing to sacrifice or invest to prevent substance abuse. A resort area, for example, may have widespread alcohol-related problems but may be reluctant to impose strict controls on how, when, and where alcoholic beverages can be consumed. A retirement community, in contrast, may be more likely to support such restrictions.

Communities also differ on selecting populations targeted for various types of intervention. Several East Coast cities, for example, have targeted youth drug abuse and violence with a curfew that penalizes parents whose children violate the order. A contemporary survey in Minnesota found almost no support for enforcing similar penalties on parents whose children illegally use alcohol (Wolfson *et al.*, 1992).

These differences in community response are not based on differences in commitment to substance abuse as a serious issue. Most Americans claim to want more efforts to prevent drug use. They disagree, however, on how much these efforts should cost, on who should pay for them, and on which forms of drug abuse demand priority attention.

Each community ultimately decides how investments in substance abuse prevention should be made. Such decisions are based at least in part on how prevention can be sustained politically and fiscally. Another element in the decision is the local incidence of specific drug problems. It is wasteful to spend limited resources on a problem that barely exists in the community; on the other hand, selecting an unpopular prevention strategy risks turning substance abuse into a political football.

Some people want to avoid these hard questions by proposing to achieve "a drug-free community," meaning a community that solves all substance abuse problems through the complete elimination of illegal drugs. If substance abuse resulted only from drugs brought illegally into the United States by foreign cartels, this would be an attractive and potentially valuable possibility. In fact, however, a significant amount of potentially harmful substance abuse results from the misuse of such beneficial substances as alcohol, medications, and even some household cleaning solvents. In addition, substance abuse also results from harvesting and using locally available drugs, including marijuana and peyote. As a result, whenever some people find intoxication to be pleasant or seek a quick chemical solution to an emotional problem, achieving a "drug-free community" by barring access to all potentially abused substances rarely is a plausible prevention goal.

DOING WHAT WORKS: REDUCING SPECIFIC PROBLEMS

Have communities used prevention techniques to achieve more plausible goals for reduction of substance abuse? This question is really the heart of this book—and to remove the suspense, the answer is "Yes."

During the late 1980s, the United States dramatically increased drug abuse prevention activities. Federal spending in the field leaped from less than $150 million in 1985 to over $700 million in 1989 (see Figure 1.1). This national effort concentrated on a few specific problems: cocaine use (particularly among youth), teenage alcohol use, and—to a lesser degree—drunk driving and marijuana use. During these few years, credible surveys and studies reported the following progress:

- The *lifetime* abstinence rate for alcohol and, presumably, drugs among high school seniors was stable at 7.7% (±1%) between 1977 and 1987. This core of nonusers soared to 19.6% of high school seniors in 1994 (using a slightly revised definition of "alcohol use").
- During the same years, the percentage of high school seniors who reported daily consumption of alcohol dropped from 4.8 to 2.5%.
- From 1976 through 1987, surveys reported that most high school seniors had tried marijuana. By 1994, 61.8% of high school seniors indicated that they had *never* used the drug.
- The rate of high school seniors using cocaine during the past year dropped from 10% in 1987 to 3.5% in 1994.[1]
- The rate of cocaine use among juvenile arrestees in New York City fell from 69% in 1987 to 17% in 1993 (Golub & Johnson, 1994).
- A national study comparing drinking patterns in 1984 and 1990 reported that the percentage of men aged 18 to 39 years who reported drinking

---

[1] The above statistics are derived from Johnston, O'Malley, and Bachman (1995).

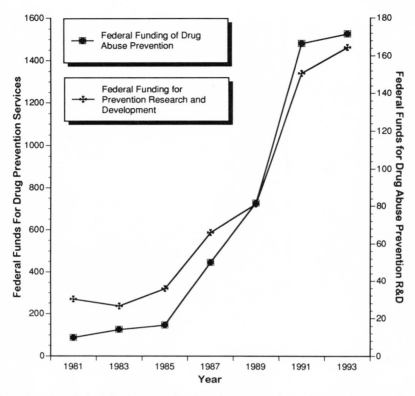

Figure 1.1. Growth in federal support for drug abuse prevention and prevention research and development, 1981–1993. Source: Executive Office of the President, Office of Management and Budget. (1993, April). *Federal drug control funding FY 1994 budget summary.* Washington, DC: Office of Management and Budget, April 1983.

    five or more drinks on a recent occasion was halved from 15.2% to under 8% (Midanik & Clark, 1994).
- Annual alcohol-related traffic deaths reported by the National Highway Transportation Safety Administration declined 28% from 24,045 in 1986 to fewer than 17,500 in 1993.

Some of this progress resulted from the application of theory to the practice of drug abuse prevention. Theory-building has been particularly strong in developing models for adolescent drug use. For example, scientists found that adolescents who are frequently truant also are most likely to perform poorly in school, while poor schoolwork, in turn, is linked to risk for drug use at an early age.

Better knowledge of the complex relationship among risk and protective factors and their influence on behavior helps guide effective prevention (e.g., see Hawkins, Catalano, & Miller, 1992, or Rogers & Ginzberg, 1992). Some theories in this area served as the launching pad for successful prevention efforts. Other research contributed to explanations of why some types of interventions appear to be more effective than other prevention activities.

Theory, however, is *not* practice, especially in prevention. Many effective prevention efforts were developed without a solid theoretical base. At the same time, some of the most impressive theoretical models of the origins of substance abuse are so elaborate and sophisticated that they offer no clear guidance on what actually should be done for prevention.

The practice of drug abuse prevention, like politics, can be seen as the art of the possible. What works is best determined by what has proven successful, rather than what theory predicts may be successful. The key is to match winning solutions to real-world problems and to modify them for local conditions.

DOING WHAT WORKS: FINDING WINNING SOLUTIONS

Scientists often offer a gloomy assessment of the state-of-the-art of preventing drug problems. In 1993, for example, the authors of the National Academy of Sciences review on the subject declared,

> On balance, we conclude that no drug abuse prevention strategies have been adequately evaluated and found to be reliably effective, in all cases, with all groups....Some prevention strategies have been evaluated sufficiently to conclude that they are *not* widely effective. The will to believe on the part of implementers and program sponsors alike seems stronger than the evidence. (Gerstein & Green, 1993, pp. 3–4)

Such statements lead some people to suspect that all drug abuse prevention efforts fail. The situation is not improved when politicians and attack journalists highlight a handful of programs that spend drug abuse prevention funds to repave jogging tracks or take gang members to an amusement park. Faced with such examples, community leaders might be persuaded that drug abuse prevention merely wastes money on good intentions.

Scientific skepticism does not alter the fact that prevention repeatedly has been shown to reduce drug problems. When evaluators report that prevention activities are not "reliably effective, in all cases, with all groups," they merely restate the obvious point that there is no "magic bullet" capable of reducing every type of drug abuse-related problem in every population. A similar observation could be made about prevention of most health problems.

Cynical horror stories depicting waste in prevention also need to be placed in context. Until 1986 government support to drug abuse prevention was very limited. Concerned citizens at the local level, rather than government, were the driving force behind such pioneer antidrug efforts as Mothers Against Drunk Driving and Families in Action, as well as hundreds of local school-based "drug education" programs.

During the early 1980s, there was little real expertise on effective prevention. Grass-roots organizers were sometimes lucky enough to have an intuitive sense of what works. Many local prevention efforts, however, made poor choices in deciding what types of programs to offer or how to implement them. The organizers eventually found themselves defending decisions made without benefit of expert advice. It's not surprising under these circumstances that drug abuse prevention developed a reputation for wastefulness.

Today there is an extensive record of effective performance by drug abuse prevention programs. During the late 1980s, federal agencies provided the drug abuse prevention field with training and technical assistance through demonstration grants and information dissemination activities. The agencies also provided funding and resources to help state and local activities. The federal Center for Substance Abuse Prevention (CSAP) carved out a niche in addressing the difficult problems of prevention among the subset of youth and young adults at risk for abuse of cocaine and other illegal drugs:

- Children of substance-abusing parents
- Pregnant women with established histories of alcohol abuse or other drug use
- Adolescents at risk of future criminal drug involvement based on personal life history of academic failure
- Adolescents living in a community environment characterized by unusually high rates of drug use, poverty, HIV infection, and the like

In contrast, most projects funded by other federal agencies scored their successes with populations that either were not identified as "high risk" or were at risk primarily for alcohol abuse.

The massive influx of federal support transformed drug abuse prevention. Foundations and private business became interested in the field. Salaries for prevention program managers increased and a more diverse, experienced group of professionals were attracted to drug abuse prevention. Most importantly, the drug abuse prevention "revolution" of the mid-1980s led directly to serious efforts to find prevention that could prove its worth. As a result, all efforts described in this book reflect attempts to implement well-conceived prevention and rigorous evaluations.

The Anti-Drug Abuse Act of 1988 (P.L. 100–690) produced a systematic effort to review a wide variety of preventive interventions. The bill required the Secretary of Health and Human Services to "develop and conduct a structured evaluation of the different approaches utilized across the Nation to reduce alcohol and drug abuse." The authors of *Preventing Substance Abuse: Interventions That Work* directed the project team for this national structured evaluation; most of the prevention solutions described in this book were identified and reviewed for that study.[2] The majority were funded at least in part through direct grants from the federal government because federal grantors demanded at least a rudimentary outcome evaluation from the grant recipients. In contrast, prevention initiatives funded by local government or by private philanthropy seldom complete credible outcome evaluations.

DOING WHAT WORKS: THE CHANGING ROLE OF PRIMARY HEALTHCARE

Many drug abuse prevention programs operate on the assumption that many uninsured people cannot be reached through the same channels as most Americans. To a large extent, this population is defined as the working poor, with emphasis on such minority ethnic groups as African Americans, Alaska Natives, Hispanic Americans, and American Indians. Members of these groups often lack access to conventional healthcare and suffer from a larger-than-average burden of risk factors for mental health issues. In response to these conditions, community-based organizations were funded to conduct outreach among disadvantaged groups and bring them into the net of effective prevention.

The assumptions underlying these policies are being rapidly eroded by radical shifts in the healthcare delivery system. By the year 2000, perhaps three-fourths of all Americans, including uninsured women and children, will receive healthcare in a managed care environment dedicated to using any means—including prevention—to reduce clinical care costs. Another component of the transformation of the healthcare system is the establishment of subsidized private insurance coverage in several states, through public funding of insurance premiums for the poor. As a result, some states are approaching near-universal access to the private sector healthcare system. It's true that some populations will continue to encounter cultural and logistic barriers to health-

---

[2] The Appendix provides additional information on the National Structured Evaluation and its findings.

care, but even advocates for ethnic minorities are beginning to argue that the solution to this problem lies as much in educating the disenfranchised as in adapting the system.

We appear to be entering an era in which the healthcare system should have more incentives than before to support effective prevention and in which the private healthcare system is at least administratively and financially accessible to the previously uninsured. Managed care encourages private sector healthcare entities to be systematically concerned with effective prevention and willing to invest resources for this purpose. Further, the blurring between the public and private sector healthcare system reduces the public's willingness to concentrate energy on a medically marginalized population beyond the reach of the conventional healthcare system. In a society in which nearly everyone is under managed care and theoretically covered by the private healthcare system, the role of the neighborhood activist as the central player in substance abuse prevention is difficult to justify. At the same time, competing budget priorities make it more difficult to fund grants for special services for the disadvantaged.

The healthcare revolution also changed the relationship between primary care clinicians and clinical specialists, including behavioral health professionals. The earlier pay-per-service system encouraged collaboration between the two groups, encouraging access to mental health and addiction specialists for everything from prevention through treatment. The economic realities of managed healthcare discourage such access. Behavioral health practitioners, organ transplant surgeons, endocrinologists, and radiation therapists now are all experts to be used only as a last resort when the primary care system cannot respond. As a result, the primary care provider is more likely than the addiction medicine specialist to be responsible for prevention.

With new responsibility for reducing need for clinical services, the primary healthcare system needs help in identifying activities that prevent substance abuse. At the same time, because substance abuse problems are driven largely by people who do not go for help to the healthcare system, school systems and communities in general still need help in selecting community-based prevention activities that work.

This book organizes prevention efforts to help decision makers select approaches that can reduce their community's specific substance abuse problems. Each program identified in this work includes a brief description of its origin: why a prevention effort chose to implement a specific group of activities to address a specific problem. Implementation factors that are considered important for the success of the program also are included. In most cases, tables or figures that illustrate the outcomes that identified the programs as successful prevention efforts have been created. Where possible, the description concludes by identifying a contact responsible for either the creation or management of the program. This contact and the literature cited are the best potential sources for additional details on each prevention effort.

Neither the Prevention, Intervention, and Treatment Coalition for Health (PITCH) nor Conwal Incorporated, which cosponsored the preparation of this text, automatically endorses any curriculum, program, or organization described in *Practical Substance Abuse Prevention.* The examples should provide a useful starting point for considering activities and programs, but some are more appropriate than others for most communities. A local drug abuse prevention effort should be a careful consumer, making choices based on a clear understanding of prevention needs and resources.

Problem: Preventing Drug-Exposed Newborns

Since the mid-1980s, pregnant drug-abusers have been a hot topic in the substance abuse field. Both government and private funding sources have lavished resources on this population. This attention produced some very positive results. An addiction treatment system established primarily to meet the needs of male alcoholics and drug addicts has developed more resources tailored for women. Infant mortality and morbidity have decreased. Hospitals also are experiencing fewer cases of the "border baby" phenomenon in which drug-addicted mothers abandon their children at birth.

The downside of the attention to the issue is a movement among some lawmakers to punish mothers for damaging children *in utero* by abusing illegal drugs. Some states have attempted to apply special criminal sanctions to women who use crack cocaine and/or heroin while pregnant. Although this type of prosecution may give the community greater power to deter women from using drugs or to force them into care, some advocates argue that it discourages pregnant women from seeking help for a drug problem. In addition, by ignoring the more widespread damage inflicted by use of legal substances during pregnancy, criminal sanctions for cocaine and heroin use during pregnancy address only a small percentage of drug-exposed newborns.

Prevention that encourages women to avoid all of the drug use behavior that can harm a child before and after birth is less costly, less discriminatory, and probably more effective than punitive action.

DRUG-EXPOSED NEWBORNS AS A COMMUNITY PROBLEM

Women of childbearing age generally are less likely than men of the same age to use alcohol or drugs, but the differences are diminishing. According to estimates from the most recent *National Household Survey on Drug Abuse* (SAMHSA, 1995), 2.5 million women between the ages of 18 and 34 have used illegal drugs during the past 30 days; roughly 10% of these regularly use cocaine or heroin. In addition, over 4 million women of childbearing age drink alcohol at least weekly and more than 9 million smoke cigarettes.

Alcohol and tobacco use are by far the most frequent causes of substance abuse-related birth problems and birth defects. Heavy consumption of alcoholic beverages during the second trimester is the single largest preventable cause of mental retardation. Tobacco use during pregnancy is not as closely linked to long-term defects, but it contributes to low birth weight and to sudden infant death syndrome (SIDS) and infant respiratory problems.

In the popular imagination, the worst result of drug use during pregnancy is an addicted baby enduring drug withdrawal during the first hours after birth. Such cases occur mainly in pregnancies among heroin and methadone users. The more common problems during pregnancy among users of other drugs are premature labor, retarded fetal development, and very low birth weight.[1]

These conditions produce children who are insufficiently developed physically and mentally to survive without intensive medical care. The expense of providing this care to drug-exposed newborns who are not covered by any type of insurance is one of the major factors driving soaring healthcare costs in communities where many young women use drugs, cigarettes, and alcohol.

The burden to society of drug-exposed infants only begins with the costs of delivery. The children have a relatively high risk for congenital birth defects and for infection with HIV, syphilis, and other potentially crippling or fatal conditions. Children exposed to drugs in the womb tend to develop poor feeding reflexes and intermittent sleep patterns. They also are more susceptible to infectious disease and to failure to thrive symptoms.

Even when physical problems are not visible at birth, victims of fetal alcohol syndrome (FAS) and other prenatal drug exposure often are mentally and visually impaired through adulthood, adding to costs of special education and welfare. The children may later exhibit learning disabilities, including attention deficit and hyperactivity, and ultimately run a higher than average risk of becoming involved in drug use at an early age.

Scientists are uncertain which of these problems result from the physical effects of drug use on the developing child, which result from genetic inheritance, and which result from the poor parenting practices that are typical of drug- and alcohol-abusing households. Research conducted during the 1980s suggests that occasional drinking binges during pregnancy may cause more harm to the

---

[1] Two readable summaries of recent research on the effects of drugs on pregnancy are Bays, J. (1990). Substance abuse and child abuse: The impact of addiction on the child. *Pediatric Clinics of North America*, 37,881–904; and Finnegan, L. (1988). *Drugs, alcohol, pregnancy, and parenting*. London: Kluwer Academic Press.

child than exposure to even larger amounts of alcohol spread out more evenly over time (e.g., see Bonthius & West, 1989). Less is known about how different patterns of use of other drugs affect children before birth.

The bottom line is that genetics, misuse of legal substances, and parenting behavior probably all contribute to the problem of drug-exposed infants. As one cross-site study reports,

> A typical profile of a pregnant woman who uses drugs reveals a host of individual problems that collectively act as stressors on her parenting effectiveness. These problems often include low socioeconomic status; a family history of alcohol and other drug abuse, violence, and sexual abuse; a lack of access to or use of health care, including prenatal care; an increased incidence of health or psychological problems...; and a lack of a social support network to help them seek treatment for their drug dependence. (Macro International, 1993, vol. I, pp. 1-6–1-7)

The wealth of issues contributing to the problems of drug-exposed newborns explains why discouraging women from using illegal drugs during pregnancy is not a sufficient community response. Comprehensive solutions are needed to the problem of drug-exposed newborns.

Happily, the substance abuse field has produced some well-documented prevention models that clearly reduce the severity of the problems experienced by drug-exposed newborns. One source of such models was the Pregnant and Postpartum Women and Infants (PPWI) program operated by the federal Center for Substance Abuse Prevention from 1987 through 1993. PPWI grant recipients included several examples illustrating the potential of intervention among women with no immediate need for addiction treatment. The PPWI program demonstrations have been especially important for cost–benefit analysis because they quantified direct cost savings to society resulting from their services.

The four programs described in this chapter all successfully targeted major change in women's behavior during and after pregnancy. Project organizers found that women who won't avoid smoking, illegal drugs, or heavy drinking for their own health are willing to stay in prevention programs to protect their children's health.

DELAWARE DIAMOND DELIVERIES

Delaware Diamond Deliveries was a PPWI grantee project operating in the urban area that occupies the northern third of the state. Program participants were pregnant women at least 18 years old referred to the program because of a combination of low income and a history of alcohol abuse or drug use. A majority of the participants were eligible to receive Medicaid and only 5% were employed full-time at intake. The women came from a wide variety of ethnic backgrounds, community environments, and drug use patterns.

Although all of the clients had used drugs or abused alcohol, Delaware Diamond Deliveries was not a treatment program; many clients did not have drug or alcohol dependence requiring addiction treatment. Delaware Diamond Deliveries enlisted Brandywine Counseling, a local addiction treatment provider, to supply short-term residential care for program participants who needed this type of help. However, Delaware Diamond Deliveries generally relied on nonclinical education sessions to raise awareness of the impact of drugs on pregnancy among clients.

Origin

The Medical Center of Delaware delivers more than half of all live births in the state. In 1988, the Medical Center conducted blind urine screens on 385 pregnant women; 96 screens (25%) tested positive for drug use. The state Department of Health and Social Services responded by organizing a consortium of private and public agencies that included the Medical Center, the Division of Public Health, the Division of Alcoholism and Drug Abuse, Brandywine Counseling, and the Claymont Community Center. The consortium successfully sought federal grant funding to create a case management and service delivery system that would respond to the needs of 50 drug-abusing women per year.

Implementation

Delaware Diamond Deliveries's professional staff consisted of a nurse, an obstetrician/gynecologist, drug abuse specialists, and case managers. Activities included prenatal health examinations, education about the consequences of alcohol and drug abuse, general health education, training in parenting and employment skills, and case management. Delaware Diamond Deliveries emphasized the sensitivity of its care to cultural differences among the clients.

The program staff reported that traditional childbirth education classes were neither successful nor well attended by participants. Delaware Diamond Deliveries created a patient education series called "Childbirth Challenge" and developed educational comic books in response to participants' requests for "something to study" between program sessions.

Delaware Diamond Deliveries found transportation and childcare services were essential for client participation. Ninety-two per cent of the participants needed one or both of these services. A project-owned van and the use of taxi vouchers provided transportation of clients to referrals identfied by case managers. Trained volunteers provided childcare at the Delaware Medical Center used by 58% of the clients. The program management reported that on-site childcare reinforced the value of healthy children among clients.

Many PPWI programs underestimated the cost and difficulty of finding qualified professionals to make the program work. Delaware Diamond Deliveries encountered a personnel crisis during its third year when the physician member of the team severely reduced her hours and the team nurse resigned. The program filled the clinical gap from a temporary medical staffing agency before recruiting an obstetrical specialist nurse who was qualified to examine and counsel patients.

Outcome

Evaluations were conducted by the Delaware Department of Health and Social Services after 2 years of program operation. Participants had a 60% lower incidence of low-birth-weight deliveries than a matched control group. During the project's operation, all of the participants' infants achieved standard developmental milestones within 1 year of birth in spite of prenatal exposure to drugs and alcohol.

In 1992, average neonatal care costs for infants of program participants were less than 15% of the costs for infants of a comparison group of mothers with similar histories who did not participate in the program; in fact, average hospital costs for program participants and their babies were lower than those incurred by a second comparison group of privately insured, drug-abstinent patients (see Figure 2.1).

Contact

Information on Delaware Diamond Deliveries was derived from unpublished project reports submitted to the federal Center for Substance Abuse Prevention in 1990 by the Delaware Department of Health and Social Services. Although the project no longer is in operation, additional information on Delaware Diamond Deliveries is available from Joe Quimby, Division of Public Health, Blue Hen Corporate Center, 655 Bayside Drive, Suite 4B, Dover, DE 19901.

NEW START, OREGON

New Start differed from other PPWI projects in several ways. First, it was designed as a service within an existing countywide prenatal care initiative

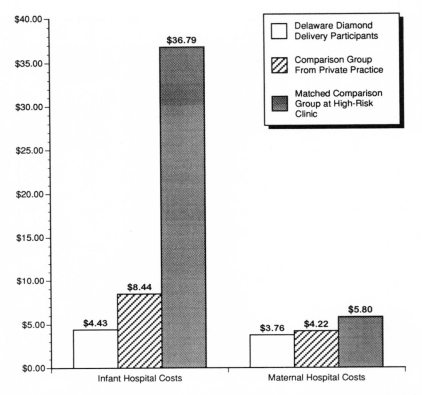

Figure 2.1. Delaware Diamond Deliveries clients and two other cohorts: average maternal and infant hospital cost data. All costs in thousands of dollars.

rather than as an independent substance abuse prevention initiative. Second, its participants were less ethnically diverse and generally younger than participants in other programs that attempted to reduce the problem of drug-exposed newborns:

- Nearly all New Start participants were low-income white women.
- Although nearly half of the participants (40%) were over 24 years old, 41% were between 20 and 24 and 19% were under 20.

Program participants were pregnant women and new mothers with a history of alcohol abuse or drug use. Slightly fewer than half (43%) were single and 40% had failed to complete high school.

─── **Origin**

During the 1980s, an increasing percentage of women in Oregon obtained inadequate prenatal care, defined as care begun during the third trimester of pregnancy or care limited to five or fewer visits prior to delivery. In 1987, the Oregon Medical Association identified seven counties in which this problem was most severe: In Lane County, home to the state capitol of Eugene, the inadequate prenatal care rate had jumped from 8.5 per 100 births in 1985 to 11 per 100 births in 1987. The Lane County Medical Society closed its physician referral service for low-income pregnant women in 1987, citing a lack of physicians willing to participate.

Lane County Comprehensive Pregnancy Services (LCCPS) was established to respond to this problem. LCCPS coordinated public health, private sector, and nonprofit services for poor pregnant women. It also directly supported a prenatal clinic at Sacred Heart General Hospital, staffed by nurse midwives with physician backup. Case management and outreach services, and interagency linkages fostered by LCCPS quickly reduced the rate of inadequate prenatal care in Lane County to the mean statewide level for Oregon.

The Lane County Perinatal Substance Abuse Task Force was one component of the LCCPS. The Task Force saw itself as a "bridge" between the providers of addiction treatment and the rest of the medical community. Traditionally, according to Task Force members, the medical community looked on pregnancy care as provided to two patients (mother and baby) while addiction treatment providers argued that the mother's drug abuse required priority attention. New Start Drug-Free Beginnings for Moms and Babies, developed in 1990 by the Task Force, attempted to replace these differing perspectives with a single case management and service system.

The PPWI grant and state aid provided most of the initial cost for New Start. Government funds were supplemented by local donations in service and kind, and by a grant from the county March of Dimes.

─── **Implementation**

Staff for the New Start program consisted of a core of full-time professionals working with volunteers in several areas. New Start eventually was directed by the Nurse Manager of the Sacred Heart Prenatal Clinic. This strengthened ties with other components of LCCPS. Other New Start staff included a social worker/case manager, a public health nurse/case manager, a volunteer services coordinator, a parenting education team with faculty from the University of Oregon Child Development Program, and an addictions counselor. The addictions counselor was responsible for educating both the clients and the professional staff of agencies to which New Start participants were referred.

In addition to case management, New Start activities for substance-abusing clients included education about the consequences of drug use, parenting skills training, and programs to develop a positive patient self-image. Trained volunteer Friend/Mentors paired with New Start participants to help them learn to manage personal finances, enroll in WIC and other benefit programs, and answer questions on parenting. Most Friend/Mentors were professional women; according to a project evaluation report, "this is a 'quiet' activity which is probably having more impact on individual behavior than many more visible programs." The program started slowly with a high rate of no-shows after the intake interview and a lack of participation in parenting education classes following delivery. Missed appointments were substantially reduced by conducting case management during home visits. A county extension service representative was eventually added to the program to provide nutritional education and meal preparation instruction. Parenting classes then included preparation of a meal served to the clients and their families, and meetings of an informal parenting support group. These extended services kept clients in contact with the program for over a year.

In addition to direct services to women, New Start established interagency linkages and conducted clinician education. Formal training sessions focused on identification and care issues of drug-affected pregnancies. The program produced a videotape presentation for use in community meetings that heightened awareness of the problem of drug-affected newborns in Lane County and encouraged volunteer support and clinician referrals.

Outcome

Program participants agreed to random drug screens as a condition for enrolling in New Start. Screen results found a pattern of relapse following delivery, but a long-term reduction or elimination of drug use over time. Attempts to include abstinence from tobacco were less successful; virtually all New Start clients who participated in a stop-smoking clinic returned to smoking after delivery.

For evaluation purposes, the New Start mothers were included in a larger group of low-income mother–infant pairs receiving prenatal care through LCCPS. A comparison of their inpatient birth-related costs with a control group who did not receive such care provided further evidence of the cost-effectiveness of such programs. As shown in Figure 2.2, mean hospital costs for the LCCPS women and their newborns were consistently lower than mean costs for the comparison group.

Contact

Information on Project New Start was derived from unpublished reports submitted to the Center for Substance Abuse Prevention in 1990–91 by LCCPS. The

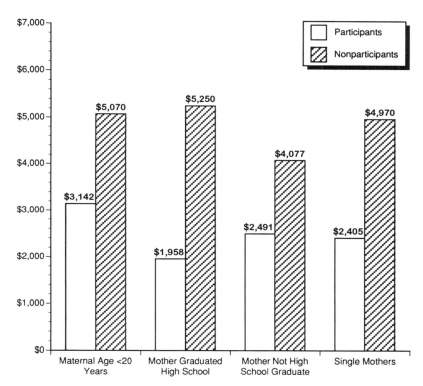

Figure 2.2. LCCPS program: hospital costs for participants and matched nonparticipants. Costs defined as mean for inpatient care for each mother during the period from admission in labor until discharge and for each infant during the period from birth until discharge.

most recent contact for the program is Joanne Lutz, Nurse Manager, New Start, 675 West Broadway, Eugene, OR 97402.

PROJECT NETWORK, OREGON

Project Network was a PPWI program in Portland, Oregon. Participants were drawn from the outpatient Emanuel Plan Clinic of Emanuel Hospital, which serves patients eligible for Medicaid and other public assistance. Unlike Delaware Diamond Deliveries and New Start, this project was designed to intervene specifically among pregnant women, aged 23 and older, with symptoms of drug dependence. Its approach also tended to be more clinical; for example, in addition to prevention activities, Project Network conducted pioneering research in using acupuncture for treatment of drug dependence among pregnant women.

Origins

Increasing drug abuse among young women in Portland contributed to sharply rising inpatient medical costs for Emanuel Hospital and Health Center, the primary obstetric/gynecological facility for a low-income neighborhood in north Portland. Project Network began in 1990 as a CSAP grant-funded project of Emanuel Hospital, in part as a means of controlling costs of delivery services. Although Multnomah County and Franciscan Enterprises helped establish transitional housing for clients, and the local March of Dimes provided a grant to develop educational materials, the project remained essentially a self-contained effort by Emanuel Hospital.

Implementation

The staff of Project Network consisted of the following full-time professionals:

- A case manager
- A clinical supervisor
- A data coordinator
- A community health nurse
- A consulting psychiatrist
- A speech pathologist
- An alcohol and drug treatment specialist
- An infant assessment/mental health specialist
- Two clinical social workers
- Two consulting pediatricians
- Four outreach workers

All clients received at least brief outpatient treatment for drug dependence. The treatment included Life Skills education and home visits to help clients organize their household. Project Network provided education about consequences of alcohol abuse and drug use, vocational and parenting training, case management, medical services, and support services to assist women in reentry into independent living.

Other activities and services varied depending on the individual client's needs. These included weekly individual and family counseling on battering, codependency, and other issues, and mental health psychotherapy, if needed. As the program gained familiarity with the clients' needs, transitional housing and increasingly elaborate child care were added to program services.

Project Network eventually became a vendor for the state mental health division, licensed to provide children and adolescent mental health services. This allowed Oregon to reimburse the program for some mental health care costs.

Like New Start, Project Network found that lack of transportation was a major barrier to serving the clients. The program obtained a 15-passenger van that shuttled the clients to addiction treatment, medical appointments, and appointments with other community agencies.

Nearly all clinic patients when Project Network was established were African-American. The hospital established a community advisory board prior to the grant application, but only to provide direction on community relations.

Outcome

The Perinatal Center at Emanuel Hospital evaluated effects of Project Network on perinatal morbidity and related costs. The evaluation compared birth outcomes, maternal hospitalization costs, and neonatal hospitalization costs among Project Network clients and 20 other nonparticipant patients who tested positive for cocaine during admission for childbirth. There were statistically significant differences regarding lower hospital costs and reduced infant morbidity among Project Network clients compared to the nonparticipant drug-using patients (see Figure 2.3).

Contact

Information on Project Network was derived from unpublished reports submitted to the federal Center for Substance Abuse Prevention in 1991 by Emanuel Hospital. The most recent contact for the program is Jeanne Sarah Cohen, LCSW, Director of Project Network, 2631 North Mississippi, Portland, OR 97227.

NATIONAL INDIAN FETAL ALCOHOL SYNDROME PREVENTION (MULTIPLE STATES)

The National Indian Fetal Alcohol Syndrome Prevention Program instituted by the Indian Health Service (IHS) faced a different series of challenges from those encountered in the CSAP PPWI programs described earlier. The objective of the program was to prevent a single type of substance abuse problem: heavy alcohol consumption during pregnancy (May & Hymbaugh, 1989).

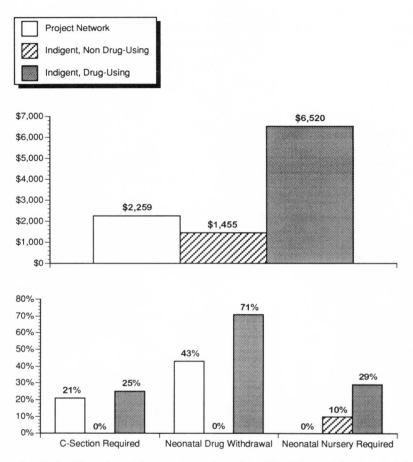

Figure 2.3. Project Network participants and two other cohorts. Hospital costs following admission for delivery versus percent of deliveries experiencing birth/neonatal care complications.

Extensive research found that few babies born to Native American women under 25 years old or in their first pregnancy showed symptoms of fetal alcohol effects. For this reason, the IHS selected schoolchildren and women in their first pregnancy as the priority targets for a program designed to stop the dangerous drinking behavior before it starts.

The scope of the program also was much larger than the PPWI projects. The Indian Fetal Alcohol Syndrome Prevention Program hoped to influence the behavior of nearly 160,000 adolescents and young women scattered among the service areas of 92 mostly rural field offices of the IHS. The program scope thus more closely resembled a statewide program than a community effort. Cultural diversity among Native Americans and intertribal differences in the incidence of FAS created additional challenges to successful implementation of the program.

Origin

The task faced by the IHS was to prevent fetal alcohol effects by influencing the small percentage of women whose use of alcohol might damage a child in the future. The IHS found that many tribes do not suffer higher rates of FAS than the general population, e.g., roughly 4 children per 1000 women of childbearing age. Among other tribes, FAS risk was 5 to 8 times greater; even in these "high incidence" tribes, however, fewer than 1 in 30 women drank alcohol frequently while pregnant.

The IHS and the All Indian Pueblo Council began the process of trying to prevent fetal alcohol effects by establishing pilot efforts in clinician training and assessment and collecting hard numbers on the extent of the problem (May & Hymbaugh, 1983). By September 1983, the IHS was ready for a national effort. It funded the effort for 26 months, and then reviewed field evaluations to determine whether women in the target population received and retained knowledge about the connection between alcohol and birth defects.

Implementation

The IHS project began prior to a national "information boom" on children of alcoholics; in 1983, factual material for lay people on FAS was still scarce. The IHS developed its own core information package with pamphlets, posters, fact sheets, and a scripted slide presentation. It also designated at least two people in each of the ten regional offices to serve as FAS resource personnel. The FAS resource personnel were trained at a 2-day conference and workshop, and given a budget for additional videotapes and slide presentations to be purchased for use in their region.

The second phase of the program consisted of training nearly 2000 people to serve as local FAS educators. This was accomplished through 8-hour workshops in 25 states, averaging more than 20 local trainees for each IHS service unit and program office. The local FAS educators included schoolteachers, nurses, alcoholism treatment specialists, and doctors. Each workshop concluded with an opportunity for all of the FAS educators from an IHS service unit to organize a local FAS Task Force and to plan a campaign to reach the target populations in their area. The FAS educators also could use the regional FAS resource personnel and could contact IHS headquarters for help in designing a public information campaign.

Some local FAS educators proved very effective. At one Arizona site, for example, the FAS educators conducted a very active community campaign that handed out materials at stores, community events, and the local sandwich shop, as well as clinics and schools. Evaluators later found that staff who had prevention included in their formal job description were most likely to report having both the time and motivation to devote their efforts to FAS education.

Outcome

May and Hymbaugh (1989) report that evaluations submitted by local program offices found that adults and youth gained a significant amount of knowledge and understanding of FAS during the 26-month trial of the National Indian Fetal Alcohol Syndrome Prevention Program. Program offices at many sites failed to evaluate whether knowledge was retained over time. In Arizona, however, evaluators using an eight-question "test" of FAS knowledge found that mean scores of both elementary and middle school students increased significantly during the study period. Montana students also indicated knowledge gain, but the changes were too small to be statistically significant (see Figure 2.4).

Each child with the severe retardation characteristic of FAS costs society nearly $1 million for special education and welfare. If the IHS program resulted in only one woman avoiding alcohol abuse during pregnancy, the program designers estimate that this national effort effectively saved three times its program cost.

Contact

More information on the project is available from Philip A. May, Ph.D., CASAA, University of New Mexico, 2350 Alamo, SE, Albuquerque, NM 87106. Dr. May is the former director of the National Indian Fetal Alcohol Syndrome Prevention Program.

GENERAL OBSERVATIONS

The four successful programs described in this chapter have several basic similarities, despite their differences in origin and activities. In each case, the program directors learned that it is crucial to make participation convenient for pregnant women. In the PPWI projects, this meant that transportation became an issue; in the Indian FAS project, the secret to success was community outreach

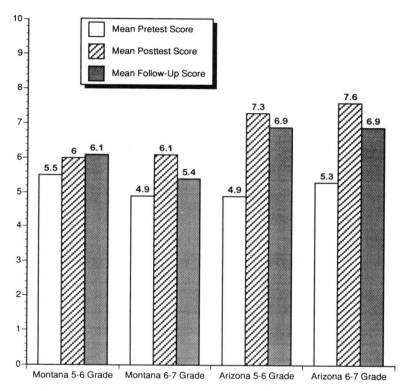

Figure 2.4. National Indian Fetal Alcohol Syndrome Prevention Program: mean scores on eight-item knowledge questionnaire at four sites. Mean change scores at both Arizona sites are statistically significant at $p < 0.001$.

that extended health education beyond the traditional confines of the clinic and social welfare program.

The program directors of the PPWI projects also found that it is difficult to get multiple agencies to cooperate so that the participants receive all the help needed for healthy, well-nurtured babies. The problem of drug-affected newborns is not solely a substance abuse issue; it is an issue of parenting effectiveness and motivation, as well as sound traditional prenatal medical care. These are aspects of prevention that some of the PPWI programs initially thought would be handled by someone else. They were wrong in this assumption, in part because other service providers often proved to be ignorant of the needs of pregnant substance abusers. In the end, successful programs realized that providing comprehensive case management, patient advocacy, and education to other service providers in the community were all part of their mission.

Finally, it must be recognized that all four of the programs were relatively expensive, in part because they required employment of costly professionals and in part because these were relatively lengthy interventions. Even the very cost-effective National Indian Fetal Alchohol Prevention Program had an impressive total price tag.

Despite good outcomes and the evidence for savings in future healthcare costs, only two of the four programs survived the expiration of their initial grant. If preventing drug-exposed infants is a serious societal priority, then some mechanism must be created to ensure that society pays for the service.

3

Problem: Prevention among Families in Trouble

Families may be the greatest potential assets in drug abuse prevention. They also may be the greatest single source of problems. The first person to introduce a child to a drug often is a family member (e.g., see, Andrews, Hops, Ary, Tildesley, & Harris, 1993). This first source is not always a parent: Research indicates that the drug use or even drug advocacy of older siblings has an independent impact on juvenile drug use that is potentially more dramatic than the better-known experiences of children of substance abusers (see Brook, Whiteman, Gordon, & Brook, 1990). Even if no one in the family abuses drugs, parenting practices and attitudes about alcohol and drugs may contribute to future drug use (Weinberg, Dielman, Mandell, & Shope,1994).

An addiction counselor discussing the changes in the field during the 1990s noted that the connection between family dysfunction and drug dependence has become a dominant theme in treating adolescents:

> It used to be, "I like to use and I don't want to stop." Now, it's "Sexually abused since age four, raped by stepfather, physically abused by another man in Mom's life." I need to be a psychiatrist to deal with substance abuse these days!

One goal of family-centered intervention in drug abuse prevention is to reduce the effects of this type of clinical situation. A second goal is to help more successful families strengthen their resilience against future drug use.

Karol Kumpfer, a creator of the Strengthening Families curriculum, cites several reasons why communities traditionally often avoided family interventions as a drug abuse prevention strategy:

- Drug use has been viewed as an individual vice rather than a family problem.
- Sociologists tended to focus on high-risk environments rather than examining family as an independent source of potential harm.

■ On a practical level, it has been less costly and logistically less complicated to contact individuals at worksites and schools than to interact
with entire families (Kumpfer, 1992).

Prevention programs are overcoming these barriers. An increasing number
of well-designed initiatives based on intervention with families show positive
effects on drug use among adolescents. Most of these programs have fewer than
300 participating families. For this reason, favorable evaluation outcomes often
are based on such a limited number of cases that it is difficult to assess what
program characteristics contribute to success. As more communities try to reduce
drug use by family intervention, the field may gain better understanding of this
area of prevention.

FAMILIES THAT NEED—AND ELUDE—HELP

When a community decides to support family intervention programs, the key
issue often is getting cooperation from the families that need help. Most forms
of substance abuse prevention involve captive audiences, e.g., schoolchildren or
employees. Families, in contrast, often succeed in eluding prevention help.
        Parents with severe social or economic problems rarely volunteer for preven-
tion activities. A study of the demographics of parent-led prevention organizations
found membership usually dominated by middle- and upper-income families who
exercised extensive parental control over their children *before* they became involved in prevention efforts. A majority of active parents also were involved in
other types of community projects (Klitzner, Gruenewald, & Bamberger, 1990).
The study concluded that low-income families, families who do not communicate
in English, and families alienated from mainstream society seldom join community
prevention programs (Klitzner, Bamberger, and Gruenewald, 1990).
        Unfortunately, the families that benefit most from family intervention are
likely to be those with significant relationship problems. Data presented at a
research meeting sponsored by the National Institute on Drug Abuse in January,
1996, concluded that individual counseling of children from troubled households
may cause relationships to deteriorate, perhaps because the child chosen for
individual help often serves as a target for family conflicts. When the child gains
coping skills from therapy, underlying tensions may remain, with family members acting out randomly against each other. Recruiting whole families for help,
in contrast, is more likely to improve underlying family dynamics and reduce
stress for all of the family (National Institute on Drug Abuse, 1996).
        Retaining families in need of services also may be a formidable challenge.
For example, the Family Circles project of the Lake Superior Ojibwe tribe found

that heavy-drinking parents reported relatively few problems with their children and quickly ended participation. The program organizers believe that alcohol-abusing parents tend to be self-involved and likely to deny both alcohol and parenting problems. The program's solution was to avoid recruiting families who were so deeply in crisis that the parent training offered would make no significant change (Allen, 1991).

The Family Circles project and other examples suggest that effective family intervention must accurately assess when problems are so severe that stronger medicine is needed. There are households that may never function effectively as a family unit. The successes described in this chapter appear to operate in a range between families that do not require long-term expert intervention and families that absolutely reject help.

FAMILY EFFECTIVENESS TRAINING, FLORIDA

Families of recent immigrants face challenges different than those of other families. Conflict between generations may be intensified when younger family members rapidly become "more American" than parents in their values, attitudes, and behavior. In a bicultural household, parents and children literally may not speak the same language. These conflicts are believed to contribute to substance abuse problems among the children of immigrants. Family Effectiveness Training responds to the challenge of bicultural families by reducing "maladaptive patterns of interaction" within the family and strengthening the family against future conflicts.

Origin

Family Effectiveness Training was developed over a period of 8 years at Miami's Spanish Family Guidance Center. The Center needed a brief intervention that could address problems in the dynamics of immigrant families while preventing future stress linked to adolescent drug use and antisocial behavior. The final stages of development and testing for Family Effectiveness Training were supported by grants from the National Institute on Drug Abuse and the Center for Substance Abuse Prevention.

Implementation

Program participants are bicultural families that either self-refer or have been referred for a behavioral or psychological evaluation of a child between the ages of 6 and 12 years. Family Effectiveness Training consists of 13 weekly sessions delivered to the entire family by a family therapist familiar with the clients' culture. The sessions vary in duration from 90 to 120 minutes and cover four major topics:

- Effective parenting skills (sessions 1–2)
- Bicultural effectiveness training (sessions 3–6)
- Family communication/conflict resolution skills (sessions 7–9)
- Drug use within the context of family functioning (sessions 10–13)

In addition to the scheduled curriculum, Family Effectiveness Training incorporates brief Strategic Family Therapy tailored to each household's needs. In some experiments using the technique, participating families also could receive occasional crisis counseling during the months after completion of Family Effectiveness Training.

Outcome

Family Effectiveness Training was evaluated in the 1980s using the sophisticated Solomon Four Group Design. This research strategy permits comparison of outcomes among two groups receiving the Family Effectiveness Training and two control groups receiving only occasional crisis counseling; the control groups received Family Effectiveness Training after completion of the experimental trial. Statistically significant improvements among program participants, compared to control families after 6 months, included:

- More functional family structures and dynamics
- Improvement in the children's behavior and social skills
- Improved self-concept among the children

Since this early trial, Family Effectiveness Training outcomes have been compared to the outcomes of individual therapy. The results presented at a 1996 expert panel of the National Institute on Drug Abuse suggest that children may achieve more rapid progress in developing coping behaviors using individual therapy, but that Family Effectiveness Training improves the functioning of the entire family and may be more effective in producing long-term change for all family members.

Contact

Additional details on Family Effectiveness Training are found in Szapocznik *et al.* (1989). Jose Szapocznik, Ph.D., the principal developer of Family Effectiveness Training, can be contacted directly at the Spanish Family Guidance Center, 1425 NW 10th Avenue, Miami, FL 33136.

STRENGTHENING BLACK FAMILIES, ALABAMA

In the Strengthening Black Families project, the creator of a nationally known family intervention program adapted its elements to meet the specific needs of single-parent, substance-abusing households in the predominantly African-American town of Selma, Alabama. In place of formal family therapy used in other programs for substance-abusing families, the Selma program provided a family skills training program that represented a potentially lower-cost intervention.

Origin

Rural Dallas County, Alabama, faced an epidemic of "imported" addiction among low-income residents in the 1980s. Young African Americans who had developed drug dependence in northern cities were returning to the community for family support while "drying out." As a result of this pattern, a relatively high rate of history of drug use was reported among African-American single mothers in publicly subsidized housing in Selma, the county seat.

Selma's Cahaba Mental Health Center sought an intervention to protect the children of these mothers from continuing the pattern of drug use. A solution was found in the Family Skills Training Program developed by Kumpfer and DeMarsh in 1981, with funding from the National Institute on Drug Abuse. This skills training formed the nucleus of the Strengthening Families Program, designed by Kumpfer and DeMarsh specifically to meet the needs of children of recovering drug users. Cahaba Mental Health Center worked with Dr. Kumpfer to modify the Strengthening Families Program for rural African-American women; the Alabama Department of Mental Health and Mental Retardation and the federal Office for Substance Abuse Prevention provided grant funding for a 4-year trial period.

Implementation

As with many programs targeting troubled families, Cahaba Mental Health Center encountered difficulty recruiting and retaining participants. Recruitment improved after initial attempts to recruit at recovery support group meetings were replaced with recruitment at such unorthodox settings as a neighborhood card party. Sixty-two families eventually participated; this seemingly small number included most low-income African-American households headed by a drug-using or recovering single mother in Selma.

Dropouts from the program were reduced through providing transportation to the community center where the sessions were held, treating all family members to dinner at the completion of the course, and offering coupons for merchandise at the end of participation. The project eventually retained 82% of the families recruited for intake.

Strengthening Black Families consists of three 14-week courses: children's skills, parent training, and family skills training. Cahaba Mental Health Center created culturally appropriate course materials written for third-grade literacy level—the typical reading standard of most parent participants. The three courses emphasize communication, social skills, and positive feedback. Mothers and 6 to 12-year-old children work together in the family skills training on play therapy, family communications, and effective discipline. The children's sessions also include peer resistance skills, problem-solving skills, and drug education.

In addition to educational sessions, Strengthening Black Families facilitators found themselves increasingly involved in referrals and service advocacy. Thus, although case management was not a planned program element, case management functions evolved over time.

Most key personnel in the Selma project held advanced professional degrees in mental health fields. Evaluators credit the competence and stability of the staff with much of the program success. By the fourth year, however, staff members reported experiencing widespread burnout. In addition, high staff costs prevented the county from operating the project after expiration of the federal grant.

Outcome

All participating mothers who had been using alcohol or other drugs at the outset of the project had significantly reduced their use by the end of the program. Perhaps more importantly, the children of participating mothers who had been most heavily involved in drug use scored significant improvements in almost every area of behavior and emotional function measured by the Achenbach Child Behavior Checklist. This improvement, in turn, would be reflected in lower intake to child counseling and mental health services, as well as greatly reduced involvement in disruptive behavior in school.

Contact

Details on the Strengthening Black Families project are found in an unpublished final report submitted by James V. Laney of the Alabama Department of Mental Health and Mental Retardation to the federal Office for Substance Abuse

Prevention in November, 1991. The final report included an evaluation by Dr. Karol Kumpfer. Dr. Kumpfer can be contacted directly on Family Skills Training and the variations of the Strengthening Families Program through the Department of Health Education, University of Utah, Salt Lake City, UT 84112.

SURVIVAL TRAINING FOR PARENTS, OHIO

Unlike the other interventions described in this chapter, Survival Training for Parents is designed to help average families reduce the stress of surviving normal adolescent changes. It follows the tradition of parenting education programs for primary prevention of drug use and other behavioral health problems.

Origin

Survival Training for Parents was developed by psychologists at the Cuyahoga Valley Counseling Center in Ohio. The creators consciously modeled the program on principles of classic Adlerian developmental psychology, with its emphasis on positive behavior, good communication, and reflective listening. Curriculum content was partly derived from Systematic Training for Effective Parenting (STEP), a program tailored for parents of older teenagers (see Dinkmeyer & McKay, 1976).

Implementation

Survival Training for Parents consists of six weekly sessions of $2\frac{1}{2}$ hours duration. The first three sessions provide information on child development and on challenges encountered by parents of adolescents. The remaining sessions use role modeling, lectures, and skill-building exercises for instruction on parenting roles and skills. In addition to the in-class exercises, Survival Training for Parents provides a handbook and homework assignments.

The training is offered to groups of parents of children 10 to 12 years old and requires at least ten participants to implement discussion and role-playing activities. A male and female faciliator are used to model the shared parenting taught in the curriculum. The parent skills training can be conducted at a wide variety of locations. Settings used include churches, libraries, and schools.

Outcome

An evaluation of the effectiveness of Survival Training for Parents was conducted among parents at two schools; only mothers volunteered to participate in

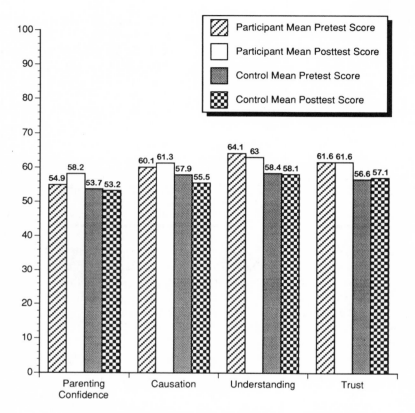

Parent Attitude Survey Categories (Hereford, 1963)

N=18

Figure 3.1. Parent survival training: change in mean scores on Hereford Parent Attitude Survey. Control/participant differences for confidence, causation, and understanding were significant at $p <$ 0.05. Source: Huhn and Zimpfer (1989), p. 315.

the experimental trials. Pre- and posttest measures of attitudes, child behavior, and family dynamics were collected from one child of each participating mother.

Figure 3.1 identifies statistically significant differences in parenting attitudes among mothers, suggesting the success of the training in influencing positive perceptions of parenting tasks and child behavior. The children of participating mothers developed more positive attitudes toward school and toward academic activities, but no other changes were measured among children at the time of the posttest. The evaluation study directors assumed that most important outcomes among children whose parents had received Survival Training for Parents would occur over time after the parents used their new skills.

Contact

Survival Training for Parents is described in greater detail in Huhn and Zimpfer (1989). Ralph P. Huhn can be contacted through the Portage Path CMHC, 340 South Broadway, Akron, Ohio 44308.

YCOSA TARGETED PREVENTION, ALABAMA

The Young Children of Substance Abusers (YCOSA) Targeted Prevention in Mobile consisted of an integrated package of home-based, family-oriented intervention and case management. All participant families included at least one parent recovering from addiction and at least one child between the ages of 13 and 20 who presented early alcohol or drug use, or a history of abuse, neglect, delinquency, severe mental health problems, or truancy. The objective of the project was to reduce the need for social services and addiction services among the children through a managed care approach to therapeutic help.

Origin

The program was developed by the Mobile Mental Health Center for the Alabama Department of Mental Health and Mental Retardation, with funding support from the federal Office for Substance Abuse Prevention.

Implementation

The primary interventions available through the Mobile YCOSA program were case management, in-home family therapy, and therapeutic foster care for the most threatening situations. Two-person teams of professional therapists made the initial family contacts and served as "gatekeepers" to the managed care. A case manager later became involved to provide continuity of care and to coordinate access to a wider range of therapeutic services. Case management usually followed a four-step sequence:

- Formal assessment of the adolescent and the others in the immediate family environment
- Development of a service plan coordinated with other agencies

- Linkage of adolescents to the service providers identified in the service plan, including advocacy for the adolescent to secure services and entitled benefits
- Regular monitoring contacts with the family

By relieving therapists of these nonclinical tasks, YCOSA permitted clinicians to concentrate on clinical issues. A case manager performed these tasks more efficiently and at lower cost, enabling case management and family supervision to continue for a year or longer beyond the end of intensive therapy.

In addition to helping the families, the project conducted community outreach presentations. These contacts improved interagency coordination and public understanding of the problems experienced by children of substance abusers. Outreach presentations also often resulted in recruitment of volunteer resources as additional referrals for the families.

Outcome

Two years after intake, adolescent clients of the YCOSA program showed a significant reduction in drug use, as measured by a standard Alcohol/Drug Use Evaluation Score (see Figure 3.2). Children in a comparison group of families who did not participate in the program tended to increase drug use. When families did not require either intensive counseling or therapeutic foster care, YCOSA's administration of case management services was associated with even greater mean reduction in adolescent drug use.

Impressive program effects also were observed on the Maladaptive Behavior Record (see Figure 3.3), where families who completed the full program showed the greatest improvement. The same finding applies to a reduction in assessed need for social services, as measured by the standard Service Utilization and Need (SUN) Score. This last measure is particularly interesting for its implication that money spent on the YCOSA program produced long-term net savings in social service and criminal justice costs.

Contact

Information on the YCOSA Targeted Prevention Project is derived primarily from a final report submitted by Marie Mello of the Mobile Mental Health Center to the federal Office for Substance Abuse Prevention in April, 1992. Marie Mello can be contacted through the Mobile Mental Health Center, 1102 Government Street, Mobile, AL 36604.

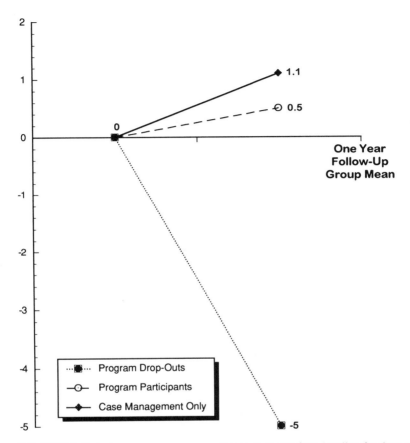

Figure 3.2. YCOSA Project: one-year mean group change in scores from baseline for drug use evaluation scores. Higher numbers indicate reduction of variety, frequency, amount, and observed consequences of substance abuse.

GENERAL OBSERVATIONS

Programs that document success with dysfunctional families, like those that were successful with pregnant substance abusers, tend to be relatively expensive. The Family Effectiveness Training, Strengthening Families program, and YCOSA project all demanded at least some involvement by mental health professionals. Well-meaning nonprofessionals and volunteers simply lack the training and

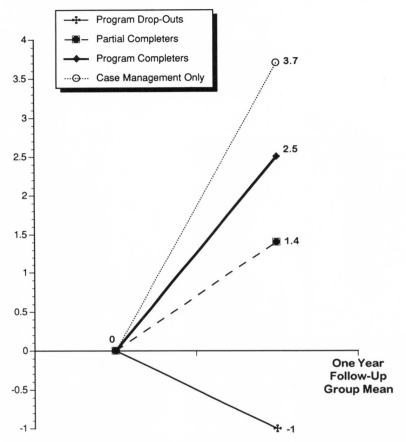

Figure 3.3. YCOSA Project: One-year mean group change in scores from baseline for (Junior) Maladaptive Behavior Record (MBR). Higher scores indicate less maladaptive behavior.

patience to sort out individual, developmental, environmental, and relationship problems that dominate the dynamics of families in trouble. The two examples from Alabama demonstrate that it is still possible to minimize the involvement of professional family therapists and use less-specialized personnel.

Working with such families is no picnic. The members of the household may rationalize and defend behavior that is clearly destructive to the family and to the children. They may resent and attack the people who are trying to help. Under these conditions, it is not surprising that turnover and burnout among program staff tend to be high, requiring significant investment in recruiting new staff, maintaining morale, and preserving the integrity of the intervention among replacement personnel.

Researchers found that dysfunctional families are most likely to withdraw from an offer of help that focuses on parent training alone (e.g., see Prinz & Miller, 1994). Less dysfunctional families—in other words, families facing "normal" problems—seem more likely to voluntarily remain in family interventions and to benefit from the less intensive services offered by such parent-focused programs as Survival Training for Parents.

The fundamental issue with all of the examples described in this chapter is uncertainty about long-term effects. Behavioral researchers are convinced that the possibility of addiction, criminal careers, adolescent pregnancy, and other social and mental health problems is increased by childhood experiences in a family in trouble. There is less certainty about whether the relatively brief interventions outlined here make a difference that can be observed years after the end of the program. It is possible, on the one hand, that many families who were sufficiently motivated to complete these preventive interventions also were families healthy enough to work out their problems unaided. On the other hand, improved retention of more dysfunctional families make this possibility less likely with each advance in family intervention techniques.

The fact that scientists have not documented a large array of long-term outcomes from family intervention does not mean that these programs are ineffective. In fact, family intervention may be very effective and the short-term benefits suggest that families receive significant help from family therapy, parent training, and case management. Moreover, the potential cost of failing to do something for these families is so high that even modest success probably is worth the expense of the prevention programs. The most recent statistics tell us that much of the increase in adolescent drug use observed during the mid-1990s is being driven by children from such families who have begun using marijuana, cocaine, and even heroin before entering eighth grade.

With this in mind, it is worth noting that private primary health care providers in the managed care environment have begun to express an interest in a "whole family" approach to behavioral healthcare. In 1995, a few health maintenance organizations (HMOs) were experimenting with projects in such areas as family stress reduction and improved parenting techniques. In one example, the Group Health Cooperative of Puget Sound, serving one-fourth of the insured population in the Seattle metropolitan area, received a grant to develop a child abuse prevention intervention.

More U.S. families, including single-parent households on Medicaid, are becoming enrolled in healthcare services operating under managed care. Under these conditions, private sector clinicians and administrators responsible for the care of the children of these households may find competitive advantages in identifying and intervening early with families in trouble. The alternative is waiting—waiting until family problems generate clinical treatment costs.

Problem: Prevention among Young Children

The idea of drug abuse prevention operating from kindergarten through 12th grade is popular and attractive. Few prevention initiatives among young children, however, show success in either reducing substance abuse or affecting risk and protective factors associated with drug use. The examples of prevention presented in this chapter demonstrate that positive results *can* be attained by programs for young children. Some programs documented short-term reduction in the incidence of adolescent tobacco or alcohol use. Other programs influenced the risk and protective factors associated with early use of alcohol and drugs. The achievements of even the best programs for young children, however, appear modest in comparison to the outcomes recorded by preventive interventions applied to older age groups.

Ultimately, any investment in early childhood drug abuse prevention may reflect faith rather than science. For example, would any curriculum developed during the Eisenhower years prepared kindergarteners for the drug abuse temptations they faced as college students 15 years later? There is no certain answer. Similarly, we can hope rather than know that today's early childhood prevention efforts are appropriate for the drug abuse problems of the next century.

WHAT KINDS OF INTERVENTION CAN YOUNG CHILDREN USE?

Schools and communities that invest in drug abuse prevention among young children usually choose from among five general strategies: problem identification/referral, early drug/health education, decision skills, alternative activities, and mental health promotion.

Problem identification/referral finds children at risk for early mental health and drug abuse problems. The process should result in a family intervention (such as those described in Chapter 3). Problem identification thus addresses the needs of children who have the most serious problems and who are most likely to end up in addiction treatment or juvenile court. Some disadvantages of the approach are that it may stigmatize families, it may produce "false positives," and it may identify more cases than can be handled by the family intervention process. In addition, it doesn't offer much for most children other than reducing the chance that they will attend school with untreated juvenile sociopaths.

Early drug/health education uses children's natural curiosity about the human body to teach responsibility for health, including saying "no" to drugs. The learning style of young children limits the depth of information that can be conveyed. Further, classroom lessons among young children tend to be less influential than direct observation of alcohol- or drug-related behavior. Siblings or parents who use alcohol or other drugs without apparent harm may damage the credibility of hours of elementary school drug education.

Early decision skills curricula try to prepare young children for choices they eventually make about drug use and other behaviors. Early childhood prevention efforts that focus on decision skills discuss mass media and other influences that detract from good choices. Decision skills have the advantage of wide application to choices in addition to alcohol and drug use. However, young children often may not experience real-life situations in which they can practice these skills.

Alternative activities provide access to drug-free recreation or cultural programs that give children "something better to do" than drugs. Some re-searchers question whether such activities have any prevention value: There is no strong evidence that boredom is an important contributor to early drug use. However, supervised activities are good for young children for reasons other than their alleged value in drug abuse prevention.

Early mental health promotion efforts take many forms. The least sophis-ticated focus on self-esteem (see more extensive discussion on self-esteem in Chapter 12). Other efforts involve more elaborate models of the relationship between mental health and drug use. A few programs concentrate on coping skills that apply to a variety of emotional states. These coping skills include stress management, values clarification, and interpersonal communication skills.

Promotion of mental health during early childhood is similar to the focus on decision skills in that the benefits apply to many life areas. For example, it is generally beneficial to teach children how to manage stress, bond with peers, and communicate emotions effectively. Instilling such traits may not prove decisive in preventing future drug use, but it is unlikely that they harm young children. If nothing else, promotion of generic mental health tends to produce more competent and better-adjusted teenagers.

Mental health promotion may be implemented for young children without mentioning drugs but not without mentioning values. Over 35 years ago, child psychologist Selma Fraiberg wrote that the highest order of mental health must include a solid and integrated value system....a delinquent may conceivably achieve the highest degree of personal satisfaction in the pursuit of his own objectives, and his adjustment to the group—the delinquent group—is as nicely worked out as you could imagine. (Fraiberg, 1959, p. 8)

The values content of mental health promotion is potentially a source of controversy that the advocates for this type of prevention for young children must be prepared to address. This potential for controversy, more than any other single factor, may prove decisive in thwarting the pursuit of mental health promotion for children.

"I'M SPECIAL" PROGRAM, NORTH CAROLINA

"I'm Special" falls loosely within the category of programs designed to reduce the risk for future substance abuse by promoting mental health. The program focuses on development of social and personal skills of third- and fourth-graders including positive self-concept and coping with emotions.

Origin

The "I'm Special" Program (ISP) was developed by The Drug Education Center, a private sector facility, with support from the Junior League of Charlotte, North Carolina. The specific objective of the Drug Education Center was to create an educational program that did not focus on unsuccessful scare tactics but relied on developmental and social control theories. ISP has operated continuously in the Charlotte/Mecklenburg area since 1978.

Implementation

The program is facilitated by classroom teachers or school health personnel during nine 50-minute weekly sessions. The curriculum offers a limited amount of information on health and drug use through videotapes and classroom lectures.

Outcome

A multiyear evaluation of the program was conducted using all public school students in Mecklenburg County where ISP was originated. Comparison of former ISP participants with nonparticipants at the same grade level found statistically significant differences between the two groups overall for nearly all

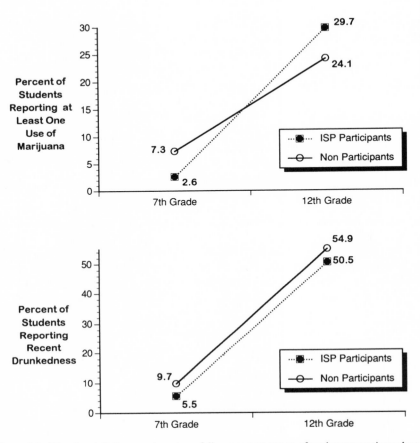

Figure 4.1. "I'm Special" Program long-term follow-up: percentage of students reporting selected substance use in 7th and 12th grades.

types of alcohol and marijuana use and other problem behaviors. However, these positive effects of ISP appeared to erode quickly after age 12 without reinforcement from a subsequent age-appropriate program. By 12th grade, no effects of the program could be identified (see Figure 4.1).

Contact

Additional details on the "I'm Special" Program and its evaluation are found in Kim, McLeod, and Shantzis (1990). The current contact for the program is Helen

Harrill, Training Coordinator, The Drug Education Center, Inc., 1117 East Morehead Street, Charlotte, NC 28204.

PRIMARY PREVENTION IMPACT FOR CAREGIVERS, FLORIDA

Rather than attempting to directly influence young children, this program provides technical assistance and training to day-care center staff and to social service personnel working with preschool populations. Improving the skills of adults who work closely with children and their family members is thought to be a cost-effective investment of scarce prevention resources.

Origin

This project and the "Smooth Sailing" curriculum used for training were developed by the Florida Alcohol and Drug Abuse Association, with federal government funding.

Implementation

The core of the Primary Prevention Impact for Caregivers is a curriculum entitled "Smooth Sailing: Caring, Modeling, and Teaching." The curriculum requires 8 hours of participant time, usually offered in two 4-hour workshops. Five principal topics are covered in the training:

- Effects of stress and coping strategies for stress among caregivers and among young children
- Techniques for improving trust and self-esteem among young children
- The nature of substance abuse
- Teaching verbal and nonverbal communication skills
- Use of rules, praise, teacher–adult interaction, and physical setting to reinforce prevention

The project organizers actively recruited facilities for training, making repeat calls when necessary. Within 3 years, the project had completed initial training to 443 day-care providers, including widely scattered Native American child-care providers of the Seminole Nation. Formal training was supplemented with technical assistance workshops on a variety of topics including nutrition, child abuse, and storytelling. The workshops were organized by the state Alcohol and Drug Abuse Association.

Revisions of the curriculum to make it user friendly to day-care teachers resulted in text that occasionally lacks scientific support, e.g., "If a mother drinks heavily while she is pregnant, her child might also be born addicted to alcohol." Such errors can be rationalized by arguing that the purpose of the curriculum is to change behavior of caregivers without necessarily making them experts on addiction.

Outcome

Despite their wide variation in literacy skills and education, nearly all day-care personnel who participated in Primary Prevention Impact for Caregivers strongly improved scores on drug information knowledge tests (Figure 4.2). In addition, participating child-care providers reported dramatic changes in the operation of their day-care centers, reducing stress for both the children and themselves.

Primary Prevention Impact for Caregivers did not measure outcomes among young children, in part because any significant effects on the incidence of substance abuse probably could not be observed until many years after the training.

Contact

Information on Primary Prevention Impact for Caregivers is derived from an unpublished final project report by Lesa Dixon and an unpublished evaluation report by Dan Balfour, both of which were submitted to the Center for Substance Abuse Prevention in 1991. The Smooth Sailing curriculum, including workbooks and a detailed instructor's guide, is available from the Florida Alcohol and Drug Abuse Association, 1030 East Lafayette, Tallahassee, FL 32301.

PRIME TIME, TEXAS

Prime Time is an effort to reduce serious antisocial behavior, including substance abuse and trafficking. It operates on the premise that interventions among children identified as clinically aggressive in second and third grades are more likely to succeed than intervention after behavior patterns are more stable.

Origin

The Prime Time program was developed by a research team at Texas A&M University with the support of the Hogg Foundation for Mental Health. Its basic

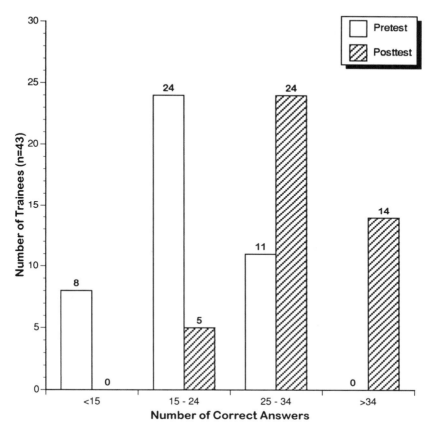

Figure 4.2. "Smooth Sailing" curriculum: change in correct answers on substance abuse issues in one preschool caregiver workshop.

premise is that supportive emotional relationships must be combined with age-appropriate training in life skills to alter the development of pathologically aggressive young children. The program designers were influenced by two explanations of the origin of antisocial behavior: social learning theory and attachment theory.

Fundamental to Prime Time's design is the belief that the school system alone cannot address the needs of young children at risk. However, waiting until the family service or juvenile justice system has jurisdiction squanders the opportunity to tackle personality problems at an early age.

Implementation

The core of Prime Time is an 18-month intervention for young children who are identified by their teachers as having symptoms of pathological aggression. The identification of the symptoms must be confirmed by a mental health professional before a child enters the program. Children selected to participate meet weekly with a trained adult mentor at their home. The parents and teacher meet monthly with a mental health consultant. After 9 months, children attend group skills training sessions in school while continuing to receive individual help.

Project organizers initially encountered several problems implementing the intervention. Some teachers were uncomfortable with the psychological focus of the consultant's comments: They preferred to discuss classroom techniques for coping with the aggressive behavior. Organizers also were concerned that group sessions with aggressive children could reinforce problems by forcing association with peers who exhibit similar antisocial behaviors (see Dishion & Andrews, 1995). Delaying group skills training until participants had several months of individual mentoring addresses this concern.

Outcome

A field experiment using Prime Time in a Texas elementary school compared results of 63 second- and third-grade students who were identified as clinically aggressive. The students were randomly assigned either to Prime Time or to a mentoring program that offered no teacher or parent consultation. The Prime Time mentors also benefited from 16 hours of formal training in child relationship skills and a weekly supervisory session with mental health professionals.

The Prime Time children averaged higher scores than the comparison group on several posttreatment measures, including peer acceptance and physical competence. A significant decline in self-reported cognitive competence among Prime Time children was ascribed to more realistic self-appraisal. The children therefore were less likely to have the sense of invulnerability that leads to unhealthy risk-taking.

Contact

The Prime Time program and its preliminary evaluated outcomes were described by Drs. Jan N. Hughes and Timothy A. Cavell in a presentation to the 103rd annual meeting of the American Psychological Association (Hughes & Cavell, 1995). Dr. Hughes can be contacted through the Department of Educational Psychology, Texas A&M University, College Station, TX 77843-4225.

SOCIAL DEVELOPMENT PROJECT, WASHINGTON

This project is similar to the Primary Prevention Impact for Caregivers in that it fosters skills among teachers and parents with only limited direct interaction with the target population of children from grades one through four. The program seeks to promote development of social bonds that are believed to protect against delinquency and drug use. Program activities include training in modified teaching practices (cooperative learning and proactive classroom management) and parenting training.

Origin

The Seattle Social Development Project was consciously designed to resolve a controversy about the origin of delinquency. Some researchers believe that socially deviant children are drawn to friendships and social ties with other children who "get in trouble." A competing view is that such children find it difficult to develop social bonds with anyone.

A team from the School of Social Work of the University of Washington tackled this issue during the early 1980s, with support from the National Institute on Drug Abuse, the Office of Juvenile Justice and Delinquency Prevention, and the Burlington Northern Foundation. They focused on long-term effects of improved "social bonding" among low-income children:

> We assumed that the levels of bonding to family and school established in childhood influence the extent to which individuals will subscribe to norms against drug use promoted by family members, school personnel, or peers enlisted in classroom drug abuse prevention programs.... All of the component interventions were selected or designed for consistency with the social development model and were aimed at promoting conditions conducive to the development of strong bonds to family, school, and prosocial peers, namely opportunities, skills and reinforcements for prosocial involvement in family and in the school classroom. (Hawkins, Catalano, Morrison, *et al.*, 1992, pp. 142–143)

Implementation

The Seattle Social Development Project operated through a combination of mandatory teacher training, voluntary parent training, and a limited amount of direct contact with students over 6 years. The teacher training required a more detailed description than can be provided here. The parent training consisted of three curriculum units:

- *Catch 'Em Being Good.* For parents of first- and second-grade students, seven sessions emphasize positive reinforcement for desired behavior and "consistent negative consequences for undesired behavior."
- *How to Help Your Child Succeed in School.* Four sessions for parents of children in the second and third grades, emphasizing parent–child communication skills.
- *Preparing for the Drug Free Years.* Five sessions on drug abuse and family conflict issues for parents of children in the fifth and sixth grades.

First-grade students received *Interpersonal Cognitive Problem Solving*, a teacher-administered curriculum to improve communication, decision-making, and conflict resolution. Sixth-grade students received 4 hours of training in skills that assist refusal of offers of drugs.

Outcome

The project tracked over 800 participating and control students for more than 5 years. In fifth grade, intervention students differed significantly from comparison group students in the percentage who had experimented with alcohol use or participated in delinquent behavior (see Figure 4.3). By sixth grade, however, statistically significant differences in substance use were observed only among girls. Former participants among sixth-grade boys were less likely to be involved in delinquent behaviors than their peers but were equally likely to engage in alcohol or tobacco use.

These findings suggest that the interventions of the Seattle Social Development Project provide protection against boys developing more serious involvement with drugs, including participating in drug distribution and sales. It is possible that the apparent boy/girl difference in substance use prevention at the end of elementary school was a temporary phenomenon caused by a sharp increase in substance use among the more rapidly maturing girls. It also is possible that social bonding may only be an important factor in the origin of drug use among girls.

Contact

The Seattle Social Development Program has generated extensive literature, including a detailed description of its early evaluations in Hawkins, von Cleve, and Catalano (1991). Dr. J. David Hawkins, the project director, can be contacted through the Social Development Research Group, University of Washington, 146 North Canal Street, Suite 211, Seattle, WA 98103.

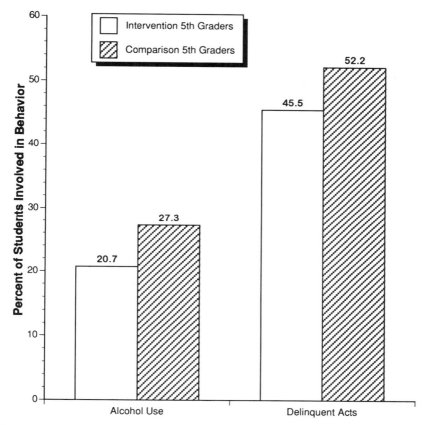

Figure 4.3. Social Development Project: percentage of fifth-graders reporting initiation of problem behaviors (intervention/comparison differences significant at $p < 0.05$).

GENERAL OBSERVATIONS

A review of programs that document positive prevention results among young children or their caregivers suggests a mismatch between society's eagerness to intervene with these children and expert knowledge about what works. Of the dozens of programs for general populations of young children reviewed, none documented impressive long-term outcomes in reduced rates of substance abuse. This was partly due to funding restrictions that prevented 5- or 10-year follow-up on the participants, but it also was partly due to the apparent erosion of program effects over time when follow-up was available.

Such programs as "I'm Special" and the curriculum of the Seattle Social Development Project remain useful even if their protective effects may be short-lived. *Very* early use of alcohol or other drugs is associated with heightened risk for eventual addiction. By delaying drug use and improving the mental and emotional status of the most vulnerable young children, these early interventions may be protecting participants against the most serious drug use problems.

A common characteristic among successful programs for elementary school-aged children is an emphasis on involving parents and other adults, such as teachers, who work closely with the participants. Organizers of two of the programs described in this chapter suggested that parents be approached to help "strengthen their children's competence" rather than fix problems. This explanation reduces the stigma of being asked to accept parent training.

A final important point about these relatively successful programs is that they lack an explicit focus on drugs. As mentioned earlier, young children either know too much about drugs from observing family members or they will not learn enough from an elementary school program to affect their rational judgment when offered drugs in high school. Instead, the generic social and decision skills offered by these programs promote behaviors that all young children should have—and that coincidentally appear to be protective against early drug use.

Problem: Preparing the Ground for Prevention in Early Adolescence

Nearly half of all junior high school students experiment with at least one use of an alcoholic beverage, an inhalant chemical, tobacco, or marijuana. It seems logical to "stay ahead of the curve" by talking to children about drugs before they are faced with the choice of using or refusing. Introducing prevention between the ages of 10 and 12 also offers convenience: Most children in that age range can be reached with prevention messages at school.

Early adolescence may also be a popular time to introduce children to the topic of drug abuse because it is a politically acceptable age. Some parents do not want outsiders exposing children younger than 10 to issues that they prefer to introduce in family discussions or church-based programs. Other parents may counter that delaying universal prevention until age 13 means that some children may be offered drugs before they receive any serious antidrug messages. Ages 10 through 12 seem to represent a "safe" compromise in which few people object that children are too young or too old to learn about drugs.

The spirit of compromise vanishes when early adolescent substance abuse prevention is evaluated. Some researchers and community leaders imply that prevention at this age should serve as a vaccination to block the "infection" of drug use for years. When prevention curricula fail to achieve such results, they may unfairly be described as a failure. The well-known 6th-grade D.A.R.E. curriculum, for example, is recurrently described as ineffective by evaluations that measure success only by behavioral effects that survive into 12th grade.

Such expectations for the effectiveness of prevention during early adolescence are as unrealistic as a belief that a visit to the dentist at age 10 ensures that children will brush their teeth after every meal until they graduate college. Both advocates and critics of prevention during early adolescence sometimes forget that the purpose of these activities should be initial preparation to an ongoing series of effective interventions. They also forget that the nature of the target population in the age group from 10 to 12 presents awesome challenges to designers of antidrug programs.

THE COMPLEXITY OF THE 5TH TO 7TH GRADE CRISIS

Early adolescence is the transition from childhood to teenaged youth. Prevention activities among this age group are trying to influence a very diverse audience in terms of emotional, mental, and physical development. Most boys and girls complete fifth grade before the onset of any physical signs of puberty. Similarly, the development of reasoning skills from simple acceptance of cause and effect to what the pioneering child psychologist Jean Piaget described as "formal operations" occurs among few fifth-grade children (Piaget, 1950). Lacking this more sophisticated form of rational thought, fifth-graders do not routinely develop the concept of situational ethics. At the same time, adult authority figures generally remain an unchallenged source of what is right and wrong.

The lack of adolescent changes in mental processes and belief systems is important for understanding fifth-graders' response to drug abuse prevention. Fifth-grade children fervently promise to be drug-free because authority figures have told them that drug use is wrong, because drug use is alien to their world, and because, as one 10-year-old explained, "it's silly to tell a teacher or a policeman that you want to try drugs." The enthusiasm for drug abstinence probably is not based on a rational assessment of the adverse effects of drug use.

By the end of the seventh grade, the typical American has undergone so many changes that he hardly resembles the child who proclaimed his promise to remain drug-free only 2 years earlier. Some of the changes are physical. Long-term changes in the U.S. diet have lowered the age of female development so that many—although not all—girls have experienced menses as well as growth spurts that may leave them taller than their mothers. At the same age, there are usually fewer obvious physical changes among boys. However, nearly all seventh-grade boys have noticed some of the hormonal changes of puberty.

More importantly, most seventh-graders have experienced changes in how they handle information. They routinely engage in advanced reasoning and hypothetical discussions. They may use "what if" propositions to explore the boundaries of the behavioral universe, such as "What if your best friend sold drugs..?", and they speculate on their reaction to situations that they don't expect to actually encounter.

Just as young children enjoy showing off their early skills of logic and memory, many older children like to use their newfound reasoning powers to challenge adults. They can imagine circumstances in which a behavior that automatically was dismissed as "bad" could be defined as "good." They also may invent an imaginary audience to supplement adults as the authoritative judges on what is right and wrong. When a sixth-grade girl says, "Everybody thinks I'm fat" and rejects parental assurance that she is normal, the girl may be either describing peer opinion or expressing her fears of the view of a critic who doesn't really exist (e.g., see Elkin & Bowen, 1979).

Despite such changes, most children at age 12 do not *routinely* face situations that seriously challenge antidrug sentiments. Fewer than one-fourth of all students complete eighth grade having used any drug other than alcohol. Unless most eighth-graders' drug refusal skills are superior to refusal skills among adults, this low rate of use indicates that few 13-year-olds have an opportunity to try these drugs. Such opportunities may come later—during or after the high school years.

These general rules do not hold for children who live in homes with many serious problems, such as a parent or older sibling addicted to drugs or a home environment where sexual abuse or child neglect are routine events. Survival may force them to develop—or at least imitate—reasoning and social skills that are inappropriate for their age. When a 10-year-old is forced to serve as the primary caregiver for two or three younger siblings, she may act "responsibly" but the price she pays may place her at risk for severe mental and emotional problems.

During the 1990s, far fewer teenagers used drugs than during the peak years of the postwar drug epidemic, but those who used frequently were more likely to have begun use before their 13th birthday (see Figure 5.1). American adolescents effectively have divided between the roughly 15% of children who live in a drug-abusing or otherwise dysfunctional household environment, and the much larger majority of children of "normal" homes. The former are likely to be experienced in drug use by eighth grade; the latter are increasingly unlikely to engage in any drug use.

The measures needed to counter the effects of a drug-abusing subculture on children are not the same measures needed to prevent drug abuse among the youth who are likely to limit their eventual experimentation with substance abuse to cigarettes, alcohol, and marijuana. This chapter and the next provide analysis of programs that have worked with the majority of adolescents and teenagers who are at lower risk for intense involvement with drugs before adulthood. Chapter 7 is devoted to programs that focus on the special needs of the "problem" youth who are likely to have begun drug use by eighth grade.

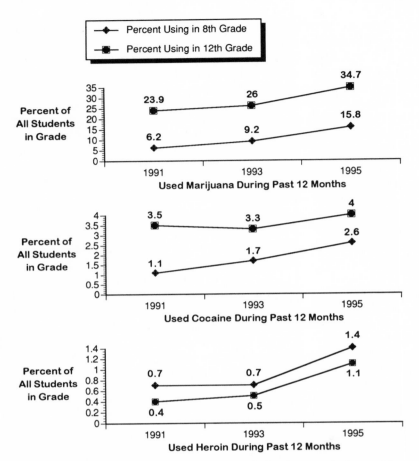

Figure 5.1. Estimated percentage of students using drugs during the past year. Source: Johnson, L. D., Bachman, J., & O'Malley, P. (1995). *Monitoring The Future Study 1995.* Washington, DC: U.S. Department of Health and Human Services.

DRUG ABUSE RESISTANCE EDUCATION (MULTISTATE)

By any measure, the Drug Abuse Resistance Education (D.A.R.E.) curriculum is the single most widely used drug abuse prevention program in the United States. It claims to reach approximately 10 million students per year through a quarter million classroom programs. Thousands of communities participate in D.A.R.E., with examples of the program identified in every state. D.A.R.E. also has become a successful export, with several foreign countries experimenting with use of the program.

The core D.A.R.E. program consists of a 17-week classroom-based curriculum administered to fifth- and sixth-grade students. All D.A.R.E. programs provide the same basic education about the consequences of alcohol and other drug abuse, safety education, and development of resistance skills and assertiveness to protect against media influence and peer pressure to use drugs. Repeat evaluations of this core curriculum in thousands of schools across the United States have made D.A.R.E. one of the most thoroughly studied drug abuse prevention efforts in the world.

Ten years after its initial development, D.A.R.E. expanded its scope to include activities for students from kindergarten through high school. Some communities have been unwilling or unable to host the "expanded" D.A.R.E. effort. Observations made about D.A.R.E. are not true for all of its variations.

Origin

The D.A.R.E. curriculum was developed in 1983 as a joint venture of the Los Angeles Police Department and the Los Angeles Unified School District. Its basic prevention components were adapted from Project SMART, a demonstration program of the University of Southern California (DeJong, 1987). Unlike Project SMART, the D.A.R.E. curriculum was designed to respond to the specific needs of African-American and Mexican-American neighborhoods in California's largest city. D.A.R.E. sought to reduce distrust of law enforcement officers in communities where the police often were viewed as an alien, racist presence. It also tried to counter the influence of drug-selling gangs.

The D.A.R.E. innovation was to use police to deliver a curriculum designed by school health personnel. In Los Angeles, D.A.R.E. enjoys the advantage of being run by a police department large enough to allow experienced officers to spend most of their time on D.A.R.E.-related activities:

> Veteran police officers with years of street experience, D.A.R.E. instructors have credibility unmatched by regular classroom teachers.... They are carefully selected by D.A.R.E.'s supervisory staff and then fully trained by health specialists from the school district. D.A.R.E. supervisors make frequent visits to monitor the instructors' performance. During the school year, instructors hold biweekly meetings to discuss and solve classroom problems. In addition, once each year, the instructors attend a week-long session to refresh their training and refine the curriculum. (DeJong, 1987, p. 200)

Most communities do not share the problems of extreme distrust of the police or widespread gang recruitment that gave rise to the D.A.R.E. curriculum. In addition, few have the resources to sustain the training, supervision, and meeting schedule that contributed to D.A.R.E.'s early success. Despite these issues, the attraction of a respected, low-cost curriculum offering law enforcement agencies a highly visible community outreach role contributes to enthusiasm for D.A.R.E. This attraction also explains why D.A.R.E. is used in towns and counties that bear no resemblance to the inner-city neighborhoods of Los Angeles.

Implementation

The D.A.R.E. sessions typically are administered during the school day to all fifth- and sixth-grade students in a school district. The 17 weekly core sessions now include the following topics:

- Nature and harmful consequences of drug use (Lessons 1 through 3)
- Resistance techniques, stress management, peer pressure, and assertiveness (Lessons 4 through 8)
- Reducing violence, critical analysis of mass media messages regarding violence and drug use, and making decisions about risk-taking behavior (Lessons 9 through 11)
- Positive role modeling, including drug- and violence-free activities and resistance to gang involvement (Lessons 12 through 14)

The D.A.R.E. curriculum includes role-playing and workbook exercises, the use of videotapes, and group discussion. Toward the end of the program, students compose essays on how they will respond when offered drugs or alcohol and to develop peer support groups. The final session awards certificates of achievement to students who complete the program.

The new "booster" sessions of D.A.R.E. provide ten more lessons in grades 7 through 9, reinforcing the core curriculum and providing drug-free alternative activities. Nine lessons in grades 10 through 12 with a reduced level of effort by the law enforcement officers, emphasize role-playing and the personal experience of students in using the resistance skills of D.A.R.E.

Outcome

All independent evaluations of D.A.R.E. have been limited to the effects of the core fifth/sixth-grade curriculum. The enhanced D.A.R.E. with booster sessions has not been in place long enough to accurately assess its long-term effectiveness.

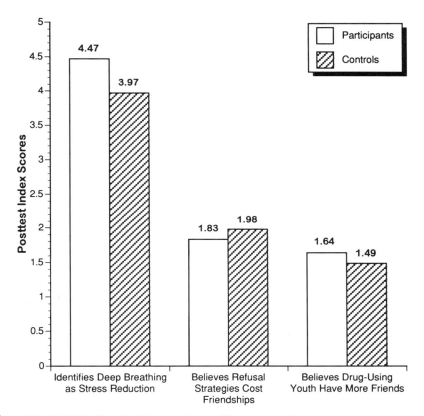

Figure 5.2. D.A.R.E. effects in Colorado: selected differences in beliefs among D.A.R.E. graduates and controls. Differences between D.A.R.E. graduates and controls are statistically significant at $p <$ 0.05 level. Higher levels of index score indicate stronger mean support for the stated belief.

Positive outcomes were reported by an evaluation conducted immediately after the 17th week of D.A.R.E. in several suburban and rural Colorado schools. Most students in both participating snd comparison schools were 11 to 12 year-olds who evidenced strong antidrug attitudes prior to implementation of D.A.R.E (Dukes, 1989).

The evaluators reported statistically significant improvement in self-concept and coping skills, as well as positive attitudes toward the police and toward abstinence. However, they also identified a statistically significant increase in the percentage of graduates who believe that drug-using teens have more friends than drug-free teenagers (see Figure 5.2).

An evaluation of D.A.R.E. in Illinois centered on videotaped observation of students in situations in which they could use the refusal skills developed through the prevention program. Three judges independently found that the percentage of students using these skills increased following exposure to D.A.R.E. The graduates also displayed other significant differences with students in control schools

- Increased likelihood to believe that peers are opposed to drug use
- Reduced likelihood of tobacco use during past 30 days (8% of D.A.R.E. graduates reported use compared to 13% of nonparticipating students)
- Positive changes in self-concept
- Greater assertiveness (Ringwalt, Curtis, & Rosenbaum, 1990)

An evaluation conducted in North Carolina used the statistical measure known as effect size to analyze the impact of D.A.R.E. on sixth-graders. Roughly 42% of the students participating in the evaluation were African-American. The researchers found no significant effects of D.A.R.E. on alcohol, tobacco, or other drug use, but the percentage of students reporting these behaviors was so small that a much larger sample would be required to document any significant differences (Ringwalt, Ennett, & Holt, 1991). Moderate-sized effects were reported for attitudes toward drugs, assertiveness, and beliefs about peer attitudes toward drugs (see Figure 5.3).

Overall, evaluations of the core D.A.R.E. curriculum find a variety of positive short-term effects among fifth- and sixth-graders, most of which apply to D.A.R.E.'s enhancement of "street smarts" rather than prevention of drug use. The 17-week program clearly contributes to favorable attitudes toward police and to a positive self-image. It is difficult to determine if D.A.R.E. influences opposition to drug use among children who express disdain for drugs and drug users before the program even begins.

There are a few undesirable impacts from D.A.R.E. The curriculum may have the adverse effect of implying that drug-using teenagers have more friends than abstinent youth and that alcohol use is equivalent to drug use. D.A.R.E. graduates also reportedly have denounced their own parents as addicts for consuming even moderate amounts of wine or beer.

In summary, the most widely used version of D.A.R.E. is a proven program that enhances "street smarts," increases resistance skills, and prepares many adolescents for drug abuse prevention. It is far from perfect and it cannot guarantee long-term abstinence from all types of substance abuse among all populations. At least part of the indifferent results achieved by D.A.R.E. among middle-class children appear to be based on the fact that D.A.R.E. was not designed for these groups. Nevertheless, no other initiative can claim better results for wholesale prevention among fifth-grade populations.

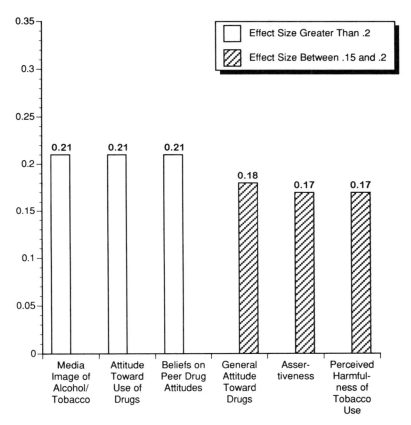

Figure 5.3. D.A.R.E. in North Carolina: comparative effect sizes for selected results. All results significant at 0.01 level. Effect sizes of less than 0.20 are generally regarded as "small"; effect sizes of 0.20 to 0.40 are generally described as "moderate."

Contact

D.A.R.E. America, P.O. Box 2090, Los Angeles, CA 90051-0090.

ADOLESCENT ALCOHOL PREVENTION TRIAL, CALIFORNIA

The Adolescent Alcohol Prevention Trial (AAPT) tested a program to counter early alcohol use through fifth-grade classroom interventions. The focus of the

AAPT was a series of experiments on the effects of variations in curriculum content on behavior and attitudes. The AAPT was not designed to generate a widely used school-based curriculum.

Origin

The AAPT was conducted by the Institute for Health Promotion and Disease Prevention of the University of Southern California, through a research grant from the National Institute on Alcohol Abuse and Alcoholism. It focused on how elements of alcohol and drug abuse prevention affect behavior. For this reason, the curriculum has three components:

- Information on the social and short-term health consequences of alcohol use
- A normative component emphasizing that many teenagers never drink alcohol, and that it is acceptable to have conservative expectations about how and when adults should consume alcoholic beverages
- A resistance training component that provides students with behavioral skills helpful to resisting social pressure to use alcohol or other drugs

The AAPT administered the information component to all students. However, during the experimental phase of the project, the researchers provided all of the curriculum to only some of the students. Other students did not receive either the resistance training or the normative component, or received only the information component.

By comparing evaluation results after exposure to partial elements of the curriculum, researchers assessed whether all of the components of the AAPT curriculum were helpful in preventing alcohol use among the adolescents.

Implementation

During initial experiments, all of the components of the fifth-grade AAPT curriculum were taught by a trained health professional. The information component consists of three 50-minute sessions, with lectures, group discussions, a videotape, and "Prevention Baseball," a question-and-answer game about the consequences of drinking. Resistance training consists of eight 50-minute sessions, including guided class discussions on the pressures to use alcohol and extensive training on appropriate responses to these pressures. The skills training in the resistance training component ranges from rehearsal of refusal behavior to extended role-playing exercises.

The normative education component also consists of eight 50-minute sessions. In this component, students conduct their own survey of peer drinking behavior and interview their parents and a nondrinking adult about appropriate and inappropriate use of alcohol. Unlike many other prevention initiatives, the AAPT curriculum does not devote time to developing self-esteem or self-image, or developing attitudes or skills that are not directly related to alcohol use and avoidance.

Outcome

Effects of the three components of the AAPT curriculum were studied among several thousand fifth-grade students in the Los Angeles suburbs. Students who received the normative education component had a more accurate perception of how much and how often peers and adults used alcohol, and what society defined as unacceptable use. They also were more likely to express conservative expectations about their own drinking behavior.

The evaluation included observing the students' reaction to an offer of beer. The percentage of students who accepted the offer following exposure to any version of the AAPT curriculum was so small that no statistically significant differences on acceptance/rejection were achieved. Instead, the analysis of the experimental outcome focused on *how* students rejected the offer of beer. Students receiving resistance skills training generally displayed a greater variety of behaviors to effectively refuse the offer of beer and expressed greater confidence in their use of the refusal skills. Students who lacked this training were more likely to respond inappropriately, such as by wordlessly shaking their head or staring at the offerer. Some researchers believe that such awkward forms of refusal produce a greater risk of eventual use, in part because a developing adolescent views them as "childish" behaviors that are not acceptable in the social situations in which teenagers may be offered alcohol.

The AAPT experiments indicate that normative education and resistance skills training both contribute to effective prevention. Combining these components of the AAPT with information on alcohol provided the best prevention mix as measured by student expectations about future drinking and their ability to effectively resist the offer of beer.

Contact

A detailed discussion of the evaluation of AAPT is found in Hansen and Graham (1991). Additional information is available from the office of William B. Hansen, Ph.D., Department of Public Health Sciences, Bowman Gray School of Medicine, Wake Forest University, Winston-Salem, NC 27157.

ALCOHOL MISUSE PREVENTION STUDY, MICHIGAN

The Alcohol Misuse Prevention Study (AMPS) uses a classroom curriculum to develop skills that help young adolescents (fifth- and sixth-grade students) resist pressures to misuse alcoholic beverages. The authors of the study observed that alcohol misuse is the single most common form of substance abuse among adolescents and young adults. They also noted that, among most populations, alcohol misuse precedes other types of drug abuse. Self-report surveys in 1995 indicate that over half of all eighth-grade students have tried alcohol compared with 20% who are estimated to have smoked marijuana.

The AMPS program was conducted in two versions. One version offers sessions during the fifth grade followed by three 45-minute "booster" sessions during the sixth grade. An alternate version begins with four sessions conducted during the sixth grade. Both versions include a further intervention in tenth grade that combines material on drinking and driving with reinforcement of the earlier curriculum.

Origin

The AMPS curriculum was developed in 1983–84 by researchers at the Department of Health Behavior and Health Education of the University of Michigan School of Public Health. It was designed to test assumptions from a theoretical model explaining adolescent alcohol misuse, and to determine whether the rate of increase of alcohol misuse among adolescents could be affected by a school-based prevention curriculum. Support for the study was provided by the National Institute on Alcohol Abuse and Alcoholism.

The model of alcohol misuse in AMPS assumes that ignorance of the effects of alcohol use is not a major influence on adolescent drinking behavior. As a result, traditional health education techniques play a minor role in AMPS with the curriculum providing minimal information about alcohol and its effects. Instead, the AMPS program concentrates on susceptibility to peer pressure, increasing student sense of responsibility and control over their own health, and development of positive self-image.

Implementation

The AMPS curriculum provides only 3 hours of total student exposure during the first year (compared with at least 14 hours of exposure to D.A.R.E.'s core curriculum). The curriculum is provided in the students' normal classes within the confines of 45-minute class periods. Videotapes, written hand-outs, student activity sheets, and role-playing exercises are incorporated in the curriculum.

During the fourth session, students are videotaped refusing an offer of a drink in hypothetical situations and then have the opportunity to see themselves exercising refusal skills. During the second year, three 45-minute "booster" sessions reinforce material from the first year.

Outcome

An evaluation of the AMPS curriculum was conducted among 1400 students from six school districts in southeastern Michigan. Each school selected for AMPS was compared with a school that received no program but was similar in socioeconomic, ethnic, and scholastic variables.

The students in the participating and nonparticipating schools were divided into three groups on the basis of drinking behavior: nondrinkers, students who used alcohol in a family context, and students who used alcoholic beverages without their parents' knowledge.

Three years after the first exposure to the curriculum, evaluators found statistically significant differences between participating and nonparticipating students in drinking behavior when:

1	The AMPS curriculum was introduced in sixth grade, *and*
2	Students drank alcohol without parent permission *before* exposure to AMPS

Other students who began receiving the curriculum in sixth grade showed no measurable behavioral effects from exposure to the curriculum (see Figure 5.4).

Students who first received the AMPS curriculum in fifth grade appeared to be slightly less likely than nonparticipants to engage in alcohol misuse 3 years later. The differences, however, were too small to be statistically significant.

The AMPS outcomes demonstrate that a school-based prevention curriculum can produce lower rates of teenage alcohol misuse. The program's effects appear to be influenced by the students' age and previous drinking experience. Students with prior drinking experience are more likely to benefit from the program than children who have never tasted alcoholic beverages. In contrast, the students who had no alcohol experience by sixth grade were unlikely to report alcohol misuse 3 years later, even if they hadn't received AMPS.

The AMPS results also suggest that some prevention curricula may perform better when implementation is delayed until students are old enough to be realistically concerned about substance abuse. Because AMPS worked best in reducing alcohol misuse among students who already experienced some alcohol

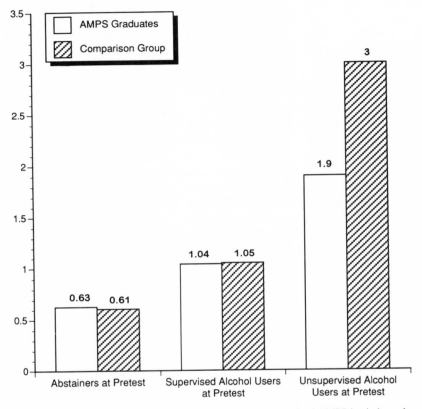

Figure 5.4. AMPS: alcohol problem index among students who received AMPS in sixth-grade and comparison group.

use, the curriculum appears to be more effective when introduced in the sixth grade, after most potential abusers have taken their first unsupervised drink.

Contact

A detailed discussion of the evaluation of AMPS is found in Shope, Copeland, Maharg, Dielman, and Butchart (1993). Additional information is available from Carol Loveland-Cherry, Ph.D., Alcohol Misuse Prevention Study, University of Michigan, 1006 Catherine Street, Bradford House, Ann Arbor, MI 48104.

Preventionists generally agree that a program operating among the diverse mental, physical, and emotional levels encountered during early adolescence should not attempt too much. A prevention effort that applies to sixth-grade students is attempting to influence people who range from childlike innocents who play with dolls and action figures to miniature teenagers who are obsessed about future careers and current romances. A program that proves that it reinforces existing antidrug attitudes and prepares the groundwork for focused prevention in secondary school among this potpourri of emotional, mental, and social developments must be termed a success.

Programs for 10 to 12-year-olds that succeed in affecting behavior or attitudes among large groups generally concentrate on preventing alcohol, marijuana, and tobacco use. In other words, they try to affect the types of substance abuse that are most often seen among young adolescents. The program content therefore is relevant to many children. For example, in the case of the AMPS curriculum, the program content clearly works best among students who already secretly experiment in occasional alcohol use, the most common type of substance abuse in the age group.

This success does not necessarily mean that AMPS, D.A.R.E., or the AAPT curriculum effectively address the needs of youth who are most likely to begin using less common drugs such as cocaine and heroin. In fact, as discussed earlier, it is unlikely that *any* brief classroom curriculum is the best answer for effective prevention among such children.

The other commonalities among these programs are that they do not discuss choices and they do not offer an objective assessment of the pros and cons of drug use, gang membership, or any other undesirable behavior. They do not present rational arguments to children who still view the moral universe as divided between good and evil. Instead, D.A.R.E., AMPS, and the AAPT curriculum reinforce the fifth- and sixth-graders' belief that drug use and drug dealing are morally wrong. They help students "solve" the contradiction of a friend who offers drugs by emphasizing that the friend is committing an unacceptable act and by teaching the skill of how to reject a friend's behavior without alienating the friend through childish refusal.

6

Problem: Preventing Drug Use in Secondary School

Secondary school classroom programs to prevent first use of drugs represent a small subset of adolescent substance abuse prevention efforts. Nevertheless, the perceived link between school-based programs and prevention among teenagers is very strong. Most of the public probably defines successful drug abuse prevention as "drug education" that somehow protects high school students from ever using.

This perception is at least partially justified: At least a half-dozen curricula succeed in preventing or at least delaying first use or frequent use of drugs. Nevertheless, some of the public is likely to be disappointed with these results. As with most of the interventions described in this work, the evidence suggests wide variation in how effective "drug education" can be for various problems and populations.

WHAT SCHOOL-BASED PREVENTION CAN (AND CAN'T) ACCOMPLISH

Any program—other than incarceration—that claims to ensure a drug-free high school graduating class is engaging in overkill salesmanship. Good programs with credible evaluations reduce the number of high school seniors who try marijuana or other drugs by 25 to 50%. The hypothetical example depicted in Figure 6.1 shows that such programs may result in a large number of students still using drugs. The important result of a successful effort, however, is that an increasing number of students complete high school without using any drugs.

Reduced rates of drug use, however, are only part of the benefits sought by many secondary school prevention programs. Prevention curricula often try to improve academic performance, impart conflict resolution skills, or encourage sexual abstinence. School failure, youth violence, and teenage pregnancy are

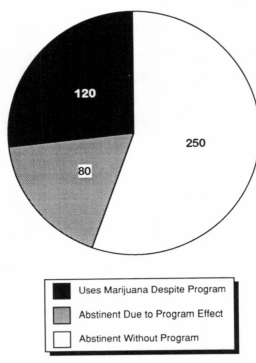

Figure 6.1. Number of students reporting marijuana use and abstinence in a hypothetical 500-member graduating class after institution of a program increasing abstinence by 40%.

seen as part of a constellation of adolescent problems that schools must address to provide a healthy environment for teenagers.

The fact that drug abuse is included among a constellation of antisocial behaviors does not mean that "generic" prevention of teenage problems is effective. Researchers note that most teenagers who use drugs also have problems in school but that some honor students also engage in drug use. Similarly, high school students who use drugs often participate in drug trafficking, but some youth gangs that regularly trade in drugs and participate in violent crimes enforce drug abstinence among their members. Although chronic mental illness and some of the other causes of antisocial behavior are associated with a wide variety of problems, attempts to use one curriculum to "cure" everything wrong with modern teenagers are probably less effective than hoping for divine intervention.

BOTVIN'S LIFE SKILLS APPROACH, NEW YORK

Dr. Gilbert Botvin of Cornell University directed the first prevention effort to credibly demonstrate long-term benefits for reduction of drug use from a curriculum implemented in school by regular classroom teachers. Botvin's program is based on an approach to prevention that emphasizes personal skills rather than drug education. It also relies on the use of "booster" sessions that extend the duration of exposure to the curriculum over several years.

Origin

Gilbert Botvin began experiments with the use of training in "Life Skills" for adolescent substance abuse prevention in 1979, with a small grant for smoking prevention from the National Institute of Child Health and Human Development. Application of the training to drug abuse continued with grants from the National Institute on Drug Abuse, the New York State Division of Substance Abuse Services, and the National Heart, Lung, and Blood Institute. The first long-term study of the effects of the curriculum was conducted in upstate New York from 1985 through 1991.

Implementation

Botvin's Life Skills curriculum focuses on social resistance skills (recognizing and coping with pressures to use harmful substances) and life skills (personal and social skills designed to cope with the challenges of adolescent transformation). These skills include techniques for developing interpersonal relationships, managing anxiety, and resisting advertising appeals. The curriculum includes very little information about the health consequences of drug use. Instead, the information component of the curriculum focuses on the decreasing social acceptability of drug use, illustrated by the documented use rates among adults and adolescents. This focus attacks the myth that "everybody" uses drugs.

The curriculum was introduced through 15 classroom sessions in seventh grade by teachers who either received a one-day training workshop from staff of Cornell University Medical College or were trained through a videotape presentation. Ten booster sessions of the curriculum are provided to the students in eighth grade and five booster sessions are provided in ninth grade, resulting in nearly 3 years of intermittent exposure to the Life Skills program.

Outcome

The Life Skills curriculum was subjected to a 6-year evaluation in upstate New York, sponsored by the National Institute on Drug Abuse (NIDA). Over 5000 youth in 56 schools who had not begun smoking by seventh grade were randomly assigned either to receive the curriculum or to receive no intervention.

After 5 years, students who had received at least 60% of the classroom sessions were significantly less likely than high school seniors from nonintervention schools to report any use of tobacco, marijuana, or alcohol during the previous 30 days. They also were less likely to report being drunk or engaging in binge drinking (Figure 6.2).

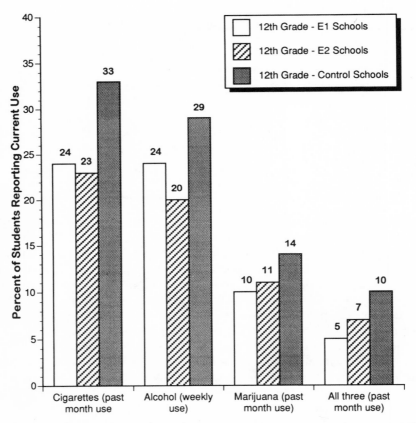

Figure 6.2. Botvin's Life Skills Program: comparison of rates of past 30 days' drug use 5 years after initial intervention (all differences significant at $p < 0.05$). E1—students exposed to at least 60% of the curriculum content in seventh through ninth grades in schools where teachers were trained via a one-day workshop. E2—students exposed to at least 60% of the curriculum content in seventh through ninth grades in schools where teachers were trained via videotape. Control—students in schools without intervention.

At this writing, the Minority Drug Abuse Prevention Center is attempting to duplicate the results of the upstate New York study among minority ethnic youth in 30 New York City schools.

Contact

There is extensive published literature on the Life Skills curriculum and the multiyear evaluation of its effects, including Botvin, Baker, Dusenbury, Botvin, and Diaz (1995). Dr. Gilbert Botvin can be contacted at Cornell University Medical College, Institute for Prevention Research, KB Room 201, 411 East 69th Street, New York, NY 10021.

DRUG RESISTANCE PROJECT, ARIZONA

The Drug Resistance Project was designed to test the relative effectiveness of various means of presenting drug abuse prevention messages. It did not accomplish this but nevertheless provided evidence that a well-designed brief intervention can have short-term effects on drug use.

Origin

Researchers at the Communication Department of Arizona State University received a grant from NIDA in the late 1980s to create and evaluate a media-based drug resistance program. One purpose of the grant was to test the effectiveness of the peer modeling technique: achieving behavior change by exhibiting model situations from the adolescents' own experiences. This is effectively a behavior modification approach that emphasizes the desired behavior (i.e., refusing drugs) rather than addressing an underlying cause of drug acceptance or refusal.

The second purpose of the grant was to examine what type of presentation was most effective for this peer modeling process. The program therefore devoted considerable effort to developing alternative formats for presenting the material.

Implementation

The Drug Resistance Project focused on presentation of the REAL (Refuse—Explain—Avoid—Leave) technique to help high school students reject offers of drugs from peers. The REAL system was incorporated into a 34-minute musical docudrama videotape called "Killing Time." The "Killing Time" script was also adapted for a stage performance format that included a live band, rear screen projection, and live actors modeling the REAL behavior in situations taken from high school students' narratives of their first drug experiences. The film or live performance can be followed by a 20-minute guided discussion period. Exposure to the entire Drug Resistance Project was limited to a 50-minute class period.

Outcome

An evaluation of the program using the alternative formats was conducted in a single high school. All classes in the school were assigned to either control or

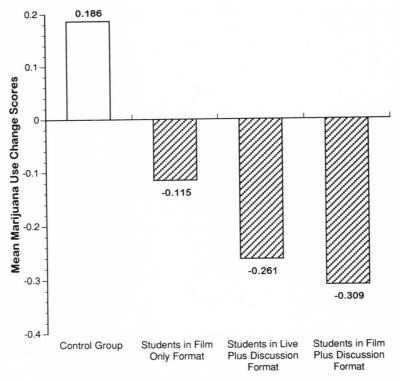

Negative Scores Indicate Reductions in Marijuana Use

Figure 6.3. Drug Resistance Project: change scores for marijuana use 30 days after implementing REAL programs.

one of the experimental format conditions: film, film and discussion, live performance, or performance and discussion.

No effects on alcohol use were observed from the program in any format, but the addition of discussion programs following the presentation of REAL produced statistically significant short-term reduction of marijuana and other drug use (see Figure 6.3, p. 76). This suggests that the refusal skills were most relevant to the needs of high school students who had already begun experimenting with some forms of substance abuse.

Contact

Information on the evaluation of the Drug Resistance Project is presented in Hecht, Corman, and Miller-Rassulo (1993). Michael L. Hecht, the project director, can be contacted at the Department of Communications, Box 871205, Arizona State University, Tempe, AZ 85287-1205.

LIONS QUEST SKILLS FOR ADOLESCENTS, OHIO

Lions Quest Skills for Adolescence is a life skills development curriculum designed to be administered in schools during a single semester in the sixth through eighth grades.

Origin

The Lions Clubs and American Express collaborated on the development of the Quest life skills curricula distributed by an autonomous organization, Quest International. Lions Quest Skills for Growing is a companion curriculum for early elementary school students.

Implementation

Topics covered in the curriculum include self-confidence, communication, coping with emotions, peer and family relations, and decision-making skills. The privately operated program can be presented to students in school or to youth participating in afterschool recreational and social clubs. The program is designed to be offered by adults with a wide range of professional background and skills.

Outcome

An evaluation of Lions Quest Skills for Adolescents was conducted in 1990–91 by Quest International, with support from the Edna McConnell Clark Foundation. For the evaluation, students in ten Detroit public schools were assigned to either experimental or comparison middle school classes. Change in drug use was not measured but the Lions Quest curriculum affected attitudes and academic skills that are believed to protect against early alcohol and drug use. These include statistically significant change for

- Student sense of control over performance
- Academic self-concept
- Language arts and mathematics grades

In the Detroit evaluation, Lions Quest participants also averaged 2.3 fewer days of school absence during the year than the comparison students. This is consistent with the improvement in academic self-concept.

Contact

Evaluation information and program descriptions of Lions Quest Skills are available from Alan Williams, Quest International, 1984 Coffman Road, P.O. Box 4850, Newark, Ohio 43023.

POSITIVE YOUTH DEVELOPMENT PROGRAM, CONNECTICUT

Positive Youth Development was a 20-session classroom curriculum for sixth- and seventh-grade students. It promoted mental health and adaptability among youth by encouraging social competence. It has since been revised and renamed the "Social Competence Promotion Program for Young Adolescents."

Origin

The Positive Youth Development Program was developed by faculty at Yale University, with funding from the State of Connecticut and two private foundations. The team first experimented with a social competence program with no substance abuse-specific content: This achieved the desired skill goals but lacked impact on substance abuse. Positive Youth Development was a revision of the curriculum that combines social competence material with coverage of substance abuse topics.

The principal developer of the program, Dr. Roger Weissberg, further revised and renamed the Positive Youth Development Program after leaving Yale University.

Implementation

Positive Youth Development Program included six curriculum units:

- Assertiveness
- Information on health and abused substances
- Problem-solving skills
- Self-esteem
- Social network skills
- Stress management

Instruction in the six units was provided by health educators in collaboration with the normal classroom teachers. Specific activities included role-play exercises as well as traditional education and homework.

Outcome

One suburban and one inner-city school in New Haven County evaluated Positive Youth Development, with half of the classes in each school randomly selected to use the curriculum (Caplan *et al.*, 1992). At completion of the program, significant effects on substance use were limited to excessive alcohol use: students in participant classes were less likely than nonparticipants to have been involved in binge drinking and to have become intoxicated. Statistically significant gains also were found in coping skills, compared to controls (see Figure 6.4).

Contact

Information on the Social Competence Promotion Program for Young Adolescents—the updated and revised version of the curriculum used in the Positive Youth Development Program—is available from Dr. Roger P. Weissberg, Department of Psychology, MC285, University of Illinois at Chicago, 11007 West Harrison, Chicago, IL 60607-7137.

PROJECT ALERT, CALIFORNIA

Project ALERT was one of the first drug abuse prevention efforts to be explicitly developed using the social influence theory of prevention of tobacco, alcohol, and marijuana use. The program focuses on resistance skills, the consequences of smoking, and personal responsibility for resistance. It also reinforces group norms against use.

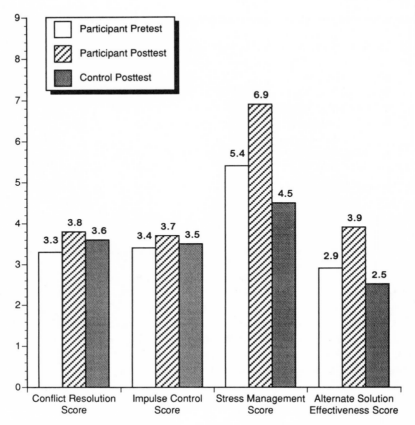

Figure 6.4. Positive Youth Development Program: mean scores for selected coping skill and social adjustment ratings.

Origin

The Conrad N. Hilton Foundation contracted with RAND Corporation in 1983 to develop and test a drug abuse prevention curriculum for secondary school students that would be more effective than earlier efforts based on transmitting information about drugs. Like D.A.R.E., the Project ALERT development included a rigorous long-term evaluation component.

Dissemination and updating of Project ALERT has been transferred to the BEST Foundation. In 1995, for example, BEST added material to the curriculum on inhalant abuse. BEST also adapted the curriculum for use with student peer leaders.

━━ **Implementation**

Project ALERT is taught in eight weekly 1-hour sessions in seventh grade with three booster sessions in eighth grade. Topics covered during the first year are:

- Motivating drug resistance (Lessons 1–2)
- Building resistance skills (Lessons 3–5)
- Reinforcing resistance motivation and skills (Lessons 6–8)

The curriculum includes role-playing and psychodrama exercises, as well as extensive material on critical analysis of advertising for alcoholic beverages and tobacco products.

━━ **Outcome**

Project ALERT was evaluated for two types of participant groups: participants who received the curriculum from teachers and peer leaders and participants who received the curriculum without peer leaders. Participants were divided on the basis of pretest results among nonusers, experimenters, and frequent users of each substance.

Through eighth grade, participants were less likely than controls to use marijuana, tobacco, or alcohol. By ninth grade, differences in cigarette and alcohol use rates between control and participant classes were not significant. Even in ninth grade, statistically significant differences in marijuana use and refusal skills remain (see Figures 6.5 and 6.6). The developers believe that these results support a second wave of prevention activities in high school to reinforce earlier programs.

━━━ **Contact**

Two good published sources on Project Alert are Ellickson and Bell (1990) and Ellickson, Bell, and Harrison (1993). The copyrighted curriculum for Project ALERT is distributed with videotapes and teacher materials by the BEST Foundation for a Drug-Free Tomorrow, 725 South Figueroa Street, Suite 1615, Los Angeles, CA 90017-2513.

━━━━━━━━━━━━━━━━━━━━━━━━━━━━━━━━━━━━ **PROJECT PRIDE, PENNSYLVANIA**

Project PRIDE is one of the older comprehensive school-based drug abuse prevention programs. It differs from most school-based programs in its wide

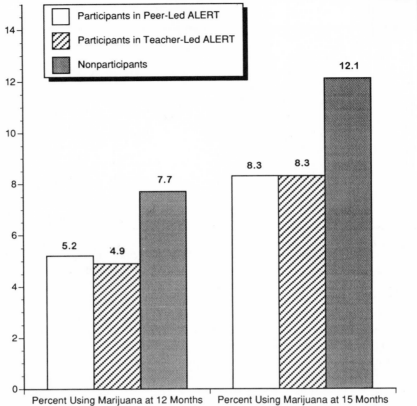

Figure 6.5. Project ALERT: percent of seventh-grade nonsmokers initiating marijuana use.

scope of activities: life skills training for students through twice-weekly small group activity sessions, teacher training in classroom communication skills and alternative teaching styles, and parenting training.

Origin

Project PRIDE (Positive Results In Drug Education) was developed by Jewish Family and Children's Service of Philadelphia in 1970. It was adopted throughout the Philadelphia public school system by 1981. PRIDE added a teen pregnancy/parenting component—Wee Care—in 1986 at four sites in the Philadelphia area. The State of Pennsylvania and individual philanthropies and

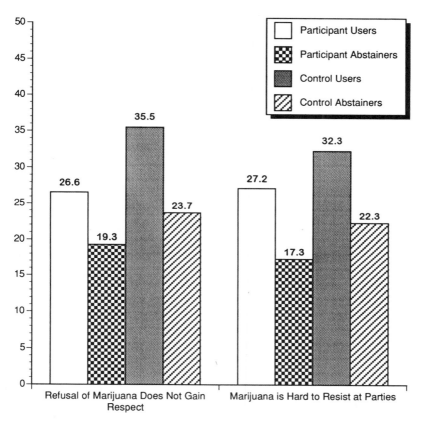

Figure 6.6. Project ALERT follow-up: percent of ninth grade students agreeing with views that encourage marijuana use. Abstainers defined as individuals who had never used marijuana at pretest; users report some experience with marijuana at pretest.

private businesses provide funding for the continued operation and development of Project PRIDE.

━━━━━━━━━━━━━━━━━ Implementation

Project PRIDE is administered by prevention specialists, who are individuals with graduate training in education, counseling, social work, psychology, or child development. The prevention specialists also are trained in the specific interventions of Project PRIDE. These specialists, rather than the classroom teachers, conduct the group activity sessions.

The group activity or "counseling" sessions for students combine informal lectures, group discussions, and role-playing and other structured exercises. Activities are designed to improve decision-making skills, relationships with peers and significant adults, and self-esteem. They also include traditional drug education.

The teacher component of Project PRIDE resembles the teacher training in the Social Development Project described in Chapter 4. Both work toward improved teacher skills in classroom communication, including use of alternative teaching styles. Unlike the Seattle project, Project PRIDE teacher workshops include material on substance abuse.

Parenting instruction available through Project PRIDE uses informal lectures, group discussions, and learning exercises to provide information on drugs, alcohol, adolescent sexuality, and parental roles. Skill components include limit-setting, conflict resolution, communication, and decision-making.

Outcome

An evaluation supported by the NIDA was conducted by Temple University, using several schools rated as "high" and "low" socioeconomic status. The effort examined the effects of PRIDE with no parent or teacher components ("passive" PRIDE), as well as the effects of the full PRIDE program (LoSciuto & Ausetts, 1988).

Project PRIDE student graduates were more likely than controls to have confidence in resistance skills. All groups increased drug use at posttest, but the passive PRIDE group had a significantly smaller mean increase in drug use scores than either the full PRIDE or the control groups (see Figure 6.7).

The evaluation also found that mean self-esteem ratings for all groups, including controls, *declined* during the study period. PRIDE students in fact showed steeper declines than controls in self-esteem, despite their comparative progress in drug resistance. This odd relationship is not unique to Project PRIDE and is discussed at greater length in Chapter 12.

Project PRIDE's effects on teachers and parents were more diffuse. Adults reported that they were impressed with the knowledge gained from participation in Project PRIDE, but pre- and posttest scores found inconsistent change in their attitudes and skills.

Contact

In addition to LoSciuto and Ausetts (1988), information on Project Pride was derived from unpublished project reports to various funding sources. The current

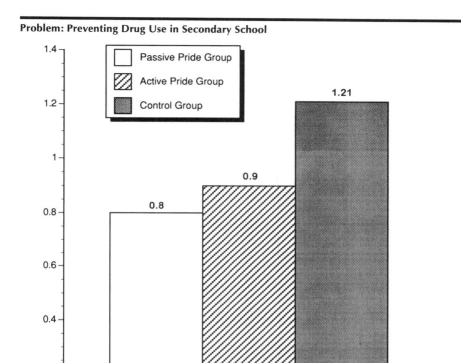

Figure 6.7. Project PRIDE: comparative increases in mean drug use index score.

director of Project Pride is Phillip Witmer of Jewish Family and Children's Service, 10125 Verree Road, Philadelphia, PA 19116.

TEENAGE HEALTH TEACHING MODULES (MULTISTATE)

Teenage Health Teaching Modules (THTM) are conducted within secondary schools for the purpose of changing student health-related knowledge, attitudes, and behaviors. Target behaviors range from reduced fried food consumption to avoidance of illegal drugs.

Origin

The THTM curriculum was developed under the auspices of the Centers for Disease Control and Prevention.

Implementation

An assessment of implementation of THTM conducted in 1987 throughout the United States found that students receiving the curriculum generally were less at risk for most target behaviors at pretest than a national sample of secondary school students (Errecart *et al.*, 1991). In effect, the THTM curriculum has been used primarily in middle- and upper-income public schools rather than communities at higher risk for chronic life-style-based health concerns.

Outcome

The 1987 evaluation found significant changes in knowledge and attitudes among junior high school participants from pretest to posttest, but no significant changes in behavior. Among senior high school students, however, participation in THTM was linked to statistically significant reduction in illegal drug use, consumption of alcohol, consumption of fried foods, and cigarette use. This association can be expressed in terms of standardized effect size (see Figure 6.8).

Contact

Information on the evaluation of THTM was derived from Errecart *et al.* (1991). Additional information on the program is available from the Information Resource Specialist, Adolescent and School Health Division, National Center for Chronic Disease Prevention and Health Promotion, Centers for Disease Control and Prevention, 4770 Buford Highway MSK32, Atlanta, GA 30341.

GENERAL OBSERVATIONS

Society's focus on peer influences among teenagers overlooks the point that most youth in secondary school are rational, thinking beings who can be influenced by presentation of accurate information about risks and consequences of behavior. To a large extent, the influence of peers in high school drug use is an example of this rationality: When a teenager becomes aware that other teenagers use drugs without suffering adverse consequences, she learns that drug use does not carry the risks she imagined as a younger child. As a result, the perception of the costs

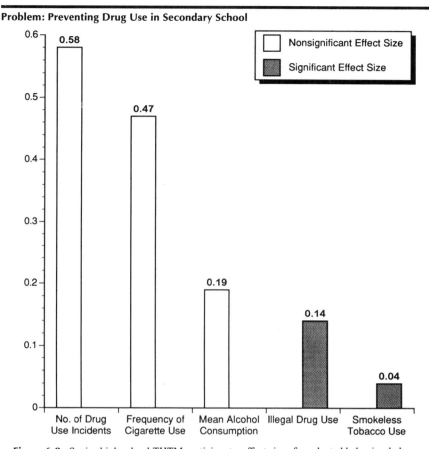

Figure 6.8. Senior high school THTM participants: effect sizes for selected behavioral change.

of alcohol and drug use diminishes while perceived potential benefits increase. For example, the reputation of some drugs to be effective aphrodisiacs probably does not influence the attitudes of fifth-grade students entering D.A.R.E., but may be very influential as a prospective benefit for would-be drug users in senior high school.

An unusual example of the impact of teenage rationality on drug use was observed in Washington, D.C. when use of the drug PCP reached epidemic levels during the 1980s. The epidemic proved short-lived: PCP use often results in obvious paranoid symptoms and the sight of young drug users arguing in public with real and imaginary companions probably was more effective in discouraging use than all of the school-based prevention efforts. Adolescents appear to have worked out their own informal cost–benefit analysis and rejected PCP—in favor of drugs with less dramatic side effects.

The programs described in this chapter seek to change the cost-and-benefit equation for teenage drug use. In some cases, they highlight "hidden" costs of drug use. In other cases, they try to affect mental health and social interaction problems that might drive teenagers to self-medicate with alcohol and other drugs. Despite these differences, they all operate on the assumption that any information presented under "drug education" must be accurate because the teenage audience is predisposed to test the credibility of anything presented by adults.

Problem: Intervening with Teenagers at Highest Risk for Addiction

Dear kindly judge, Your Honor,
My parents treat me rough.
With all their marijuana,
They won't give me a puff.

The musical *West Side Story* premiered 40 years ago, but the satiric lyrics for the song "Officer Krupke" still ring true. Throughout the comic lament, gang members portray a judge, a psychiatrist, and a social worker who listen to teenagers' descriptions of chaotic home lives, argue over diagnoses ("The problem is he's growing!/The problem is he's grown!") and then dispose of the cases by dumping them on another professional's doorstep. Bewildered and insulted, the gang members respond by attacking the closest available representative of Authority, an equally bewildered beat patrolman.

Society's handling of problem teenagers hasn't changed much during the past four decades. Governments provide potentially useful resources, but separate them by provider agency and by profession. When a teenager presents a constellation of social, mental health, economic, and academic issues associated with high rates of eventual drug addiction, it's often difficult to find any source of help interested in the whole youth. Most communities lack a coordinated response to treat the complex social conditions that make gang membership and drug use attractive to some teenagers. Even juvenile justice systems find it difficult to place enough of the youth to satisfy public concerns for security, let alone to effectively reduce the problem.

Finding appropriate resources to apply to "problem" teenagers is one of the greatest challenges facing the substance abuse field. Increasingly, the community rates of hard drug use are driven by children who begin using drugs by age 13 and may be fully addicted or experienced drug dealers before they reach their 21st birthday. Much of the progress achieved in developing classroom-based curricula that effectively reduce substance abuse among mainstream adolescents has little or no effect on preventing drug use among a population raised in an environment where drug use is pervasive and family life is either nonexistent or threatening.

"INTERVENTION" RATHER THAN PREVENTION OR TREATMENT

One reason for the difficulty in placing "problem" teenagers in prevention is a recurring debate on whether adolescents who abuse alcohol and drugs even belong in prevention programs. "Primary" prevention that discourages first use of drugs is the objective of most of the programs described in the preceding two chapters. Some supporters of primary prevention disapprove of diverting resources from preventing the first use of drugs. They argue that youth experienced in using alcohol or other drugs should receive treatment from substance abuse clinicians.

Experts from the treatment field take an opposing view: clinical treatment for "substance abuse" should focus on alcoholism and drug dependence, the conditions in which drugs or alcohol have made lasting modification to the physical structure of the brain. Although elements of clinical treatment may help less severe forms of drug abuse, addiction professionals view their services as less useful for teenagers whose sole "symptom" is occasional drug use. In fact, lack of chronic symptoms to monitor makes it difficult to know whether such "patients" are responding to care.

The evolving healthcare system in the United States favors the viewpoint of the treatment professionals. As described in Chapter 1, managed care "gate-keepers" restrict access to specialty treatment for drug abuse to patients who have clear symptoms of drug or alcohol dependence. When those symptoms are not present, treatment professionals cannot be reimbursed for the services they provide to patients. Families, schools, the court system, family health practitioners, and community groups end up with the responsibility of helping adolescents who have current drug problems other than addiction.

This chapter describes interventions that are neither prevention of first use nor treatment for drug addiction. Instead, they are interventions designed to either reduce substance use among adolescents who have already experimented with drugs and alcohol, or to improve decision-making skills, academic self-concept, and generally give adolescents a reason to believe that they can succeed in mainstream society. These interventions generally cost much less than treatment and require shorter contact than the 6 to 15 months required for treatment. They also can be conducted in a variety of settings with adult facilitators who are not necessarily costly clinical personnel. At the same time, by concentrating resources on individuals who are at relatively high risk for future drug dependence, the type of interventions described here may prove to be among society's most efficient approaches to reducing drug-related costs.

CHOICE INTERVENTION, KENTUCKY

Children Have Options In Choosing Experiences (CHOICE) centers on a 14-week group learning program to meet the needs of youth who are likely candidates for future addiction, but who are not yet alcohol- or drug-dependent.

Origin

CHOICE was instituted by the Buechel Area Neighborhoods Association of Louisville in 1988. Initially targeted at children from 10 to 19 years old, CHOICE organizers decided to concentrate on middle school: a period "when youth need lots of help in developing coping/decisionmaking skills." The CHOICE activities were modeled after a youth program that operated during the 1970s in Oakland, California, to reduce truancy rates and improve self-esteem. Start-up for CHOICE was aided by a grant from CSAP.

Implementation

CHOICE consisted of three primary activities: a school program for children referred by school counselors or the CHOICE staff, a youth offender program for children referred by the juvenile court, and community education activities for adults.

The school program centers on "self-help" groups of 7 to 12 students. CHOICE "self help" groups are adult-facilitated formats for group learning on alcohol and drug-related topics, values clarification, problem-solving, and assertiveness/refusal skills. Discussion sessions in the groups also address self-esteem, coping skills, and use of leisure time. Although there is a prescribed curriculum, the "self-help" groups enjoy considerable flexibility in using outside speakers, discussion, role-playing, and simulations. The self-help groups meet during one class period weekly for 14 weeks.

Through an agreement with the local juvenile court, CHOICE provided similar services—including participation in a 12-member afterschool "self-help" group—to youth offenders. CHOICE adult workers in the youth offender program conducted weekly meetings with staff of each client's home school, a minimum of three home visits to better understand the youth's environment, and job counseling, as needed.

In addition to youth services, CHOICE provided adult prevention education through church groups in the African-American community of Newburg. Other CHOICE community outreach activities included coordination of Project Graduation, an all-night chaperoned celebration for a Buechel area high school.

Outcome

An evaluation submitted by CHOICE to its granting agency was limited by the collection of data on program effects only 1 week after students completed participation in a "self-help" group. Short-term benefits of CHOICE participation cited in this evaluation include

- Reduced verbal aggression among 95% of the participants
- Reduction in alcohol, tobacco, or drug use reported by 78.4% of the participants
- More positive attitude toward school reported by 71% of the participants

CHOICE provided one of the first examples of a comprehensive, community-based program that used linkages to the public sector to identify and intervene with children in need of major help to resist continued drug use.

Contact

The description of CHOICE is derived primarily from unpublished final reports submitted by Buechel Area Neighborhoods Association to the Center for Substance Abuse Prevention in 1991. Additional information is available from Mary A. Bemker, CHOICE, Inc., Suite 303, 3715 Bardstown Road, Louisville, KY 40218.

DRUG PREVENTION PROJECT FOR HOMELESS AND RUNAWAY YOUTH, CONNECTICUT

Youth who have left or been forced out of their home are difficult subjects for prevention. They often leave chaotic home situations including parental addiction and family histories of psychological, physical, and sexual abuse. The staff of New Haven's Drug Prevention Project for Homeless and Runaway Youth believe that such youth learn drug use from parental modeling and the influence of adults and peers on the street. The staff also believe that the inability to retain personal possessions while homeless encourages an emphasis on instant gratification which reinforces the trend toward drug use.

Origin

The Drug Prevention Project was established in 1989 by a demonstration grant from the Administration for Children, Youth, and Families of the U.S. Department of Health and Human Services to Youth Continuum, Inc., a private nonprofit agency that has operated residential programs for youth since 1966. Youth Continuum used the funds in collaboration with the publicly funded Hill Health Center. Additional funds for residential services are received from the State of Connecticut, Office of Juvenile Justice Delinquency Prevention grants, and private donations.

Implementation

All youth of Youth Continuum's three shelters receive an extensive intake assessment, including a medical assessment and a psychological examination. They all receive mandatory weekly drug abuse education and participate in weekly interpersonal group counseling on self-worth, trust, feelings about drugs and violence encountered on the street, and related topics. Group counseling sessions often include role-playing in the form of skits written by the participants.

The youth also receive case management and service advocacy. The intake assessment can result in 45-minute individual or family counseling sessions that continue until the youth return home or are transferred to an alternative residential program. Roughly half of the youth are referred to individual counseling; fewer than 10% were referred to family counseling.

During its first year, the project had 127 participants, of whom 116 (91%) were between 13 and 17 years old. Project staff consisted of two full-time social workers and two part-time counselor aides with the equivalent of a B.S.W. degree.

Outcome

Youth entering the shelters were evaluated 6 months after intake for drug and alcohol use, and for the severity of other problems identified during the first assessment. This produced a biased sample: former residents who could not be located 6 months after intake probably include the youth who benefited least

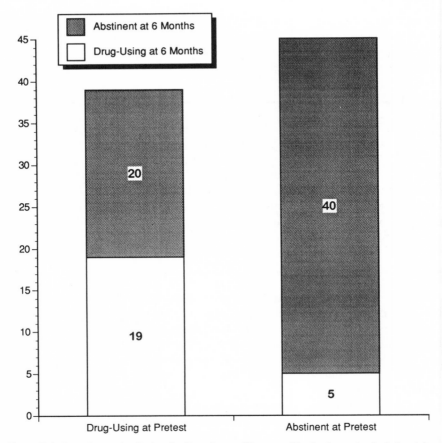

Figure 7.1. Drug Prevention Project for Homeless and Runaway Youth: change in alcohol and drug use after 6 months of participation. Data from DuBose *et al.* (1992).

from the intervention. Program assessment is further complicated by the fact that some youth were under care for less than 1 week while others participated in the program for the full year.

Among the 84 first-year participants available for recontact, the program found a net decrease in the percentage who use alcohol or other drugs (see Figure 7.1). Interviews at 6 months after intake also found significant reductions in the average severity of the most common problems encountered at intake (see Figure 7.2). Since these problems are believed to contribute to future drug use and the

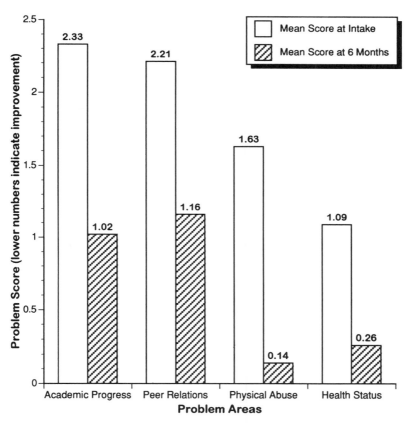

Figure 7.2. Drug Prevention Project for Homeless and Runaway Youth: change in mean severity of selected adolescent problems following participation. Data from DuBose *et al.* (1992).

onset of addiction, the success of the program in achieving these reductions may have long-term benefits for drug abstinence.

━━━━━━━━━━━━━━━━━━━━━━━━━━━━━━━━ **Contact**

Published sources of information on New Haven's Drug Prevention Project for Homeless and Runaway Youth include DuBose *et al.* (1992). Current information on Youth Continuum programs is available from Marty Lynch, Youth Continuum, Inc., 54 Meadow Street, New Haven, CT 06519.

EVERYDAY THEATER SUMMER PROGRAM, WASHINGTON, DC ━━━━━

"Alternative activities" frequently are cited as a prevention strategy for teenage drug abuse. Alternative activities consist of supervised recreation or cultural programs that replace unstructured leisure: excessive unstructured leisure time allegedly contributes to drug abuse. Most adolescent interventions based on alternative activities are not subjected to rigorous evaluation or fail to produce convincing results. As a result, many scientists have questioned whether such programs contribute to substance abuse prevention.

The Summer Program of Washington, DC's nonprofit Everyday Theater is a partial exception to this rule. Although evaluation methodology applied to this project was less rigorous than most outcome studies described in this book, the program was able to demonstrate at least short-term effects on behavior.

Origin ━━

In spring 1993, Everyday Theater used a CSAP grant to establish a theater arts/prevention collaboration with Drug Abuse Training Associates, Inc. The first efforts—a Day Program at City Lights Alternative high school and an Afterschool Program at a junior high school—produced disappointing evaluation results. A Summer Theater program for youth identified by the juvenile justice system as involved in the drug trade was then instituted with modifications based on the experience of these earlier efforts.

Implementation ━━

Eighteen youth ranging in age from 12 to 19 were recruited for the Summer Program from the juvenile justice system. The Summer Program provided an unusually intensive intervention, with participants devoting 6 or more hours daily to play rehearsals, instruction on theater arts and stagecraft, and group discussions on self-worth, alcohol and drug abuse, and responses to cultural stereotypes. The program directors view discussions on stereotypes as important because they believe drug abuse among African Americans "is related to the stress of coping with negative cultural [racist] messages."

At the end of the 6 weeks of the Summer Program, the youth participated in three performances of a completed play for community members, family, and friends. Some of the youth continued with Everyday Theater after the conclusion of the Summer Program. Three individuals were cut from the program: two for fighting, and one for attempting to assault another participant with a firearm.

The organizers of Everyday Theater emphasize that the absence of a professional counselor was a significant problem during the first year of the

Summer Program. A professional counselor could have better addressed delinquent behavior, provided training on working with the youth, and helped to manage the stress levels among the semiprofessionals of the theater company,

> Since the ensemble members are not professional counselors, they cannot always be effective in various situations. The ensemble need bimonthly training on a continual basis. (Faulk & Delaney, 1993, p. 2)

Outcome

Direct observation of the participants confirmed improved attitudes toward cooperation, including timely school attendance and reduced verbal attacks. Self-reports from the participants indicated varied effects on drug and alcohol use by the end of the program, with participants from the most heavily drug-involved families reporting significant average reduction in use.

Contact

Information on Everyday Theater programs is derived from unpublished project reports submitted to CSAP during the late 1980s and early 1990s. Current information on the programs is available from Ralph Faulk, Executive Director, Everyday Theater, P.O. Box 70570, Washington, DC 20024.

FRIENDLY PEERsuasion (MULTIPLE SITES)

Friendly PEERsuasion is a curriculum to reduce or prevent alcohol and other drug use among girls aged 11 to 14 identified at elevated risk for drug use, e.g., because of long periods of unsupervised "latchkey" status.

Origin

The Friendly PEERsuasion curriculum was developed by Girls Incorporated (formerly Girls Clubs of America), with funding from the William T. Grant Foundation and CSAP.

Implementation

The curriculum consists of 13 sessions provided as an in-school program or as afterschool programs either in a school setting or in local Girls Club facilities. The sessions train older adolescent girls to serve as peer mentors to younger girls.

The older girls, given this responsibility, are expected to identify more with the values and antidrug attitudes of the adult staff than with drug-using peers. In essence, the theory is that girls who are prepared to teach young children to avoid drugs would themselves be more likely to avoid drugs. After the training, the participants are organized in two- and three-member teams to conduct 30-minute antidrug programs among younger children in school settings.

A significant amount of the curriculum is devoted to educational activities, including information on the consequences of using specific drugs. Most of PEERsuasion, however, takes the form of role-playing exercises emphasizing resistance to media and peer pressure, and training in communication skills and stress management. One exercise, for example, consists of the participants tossing a large piece of yarn from girl to girl, with the tosser describing an event that causes stress, such as a little sister "telling tales" on the participant. A facilitator then uses scissors to cut the tangled web produced by the game as each participant describes a technique they can use to relieve stress.

Use of school settings apparently presents unusual challenges to the curriculum. In the Girls Club settings, for example, participation is voluntary and girls who feel uncomfortable with the program can "vote with their feet." A school setting, however, demands mandatory attendance and cooperation with school authorities, although program managers have compromised in some cases by allowing individual girls to avoid participating in specific activities.

Outcome

Sites used for evaluation were Arlington, Texas (in 1987), an African-American community in Birmingham, Alabama (1989), and ethnically mixed communities in Rapid City, South Dakota; Clearwater, Florida; and Worcester, Massachusetts (1990–91). Evaluations indicated delayed use of alcohol among younger program participants compared with age-matched nonparticipants from the same communities. For example, there were significant differences in current alcohol use between program participants and nonparticipants who reported no alcohol experience at pretest; among girls who had tried alcoholic beverages at the time of pretest, fewer PEERsuasion participants continued to drink, but these differences were not statistically significant (see Figure 7.3).

Compared with nonparticipants, PEERsuaders also were less likely to be in high-risk situations or to continue friendly relations with girls who used drugs. The project evaluation also found that retention of latchkey participants appears to be improved by conducting the program in school facilities rather than in the community-based Girls Incorporated facility.

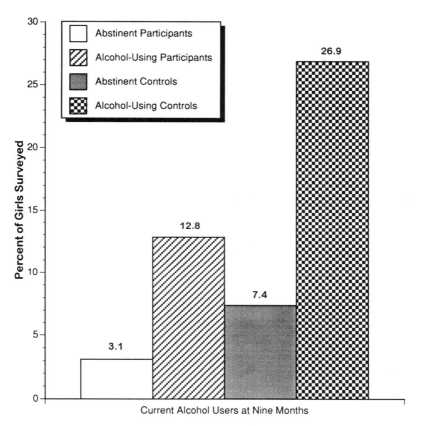

Figure 7.3. Friendly PEERsuasion: comparison of current alcohol use among participants and control groups.

Contact

Published sources on Friendly PEERsuasion include Chaiken (1990). Friendly PEERsuasion materials are protected by copyright. They are available from Girls Incorporated, 441 West Michigan Street, Indianapolis, IN 46202.

PEER SUPPORT RETREATS, ARIZONA

The peer support retreats of this program for junior high school students resemble brief residential therapy, followed by the formation of less structured peer support groups.

Origin

The peer support retreats were developed by Amity, Inc., a multisite nonprofit drug abuse treatment program. The retreats were funded in 1987 by CSAP to investigate the effectiveness of a brief residential intervention for improving the outcomes of young, low-income users of alcohol, tobacco, and intoxicating inhalants.

Implementation

Participants in this program are primarily Mexican-American and Native American junior high school students recruited because of a personal history of alcohol or tobacco use or on the basis of risk factors revealed in the responses to a survey administered to all seventh-grade students within the Tucson school district.

The primary component of the program is a 47-hour retreat at a former "guest ranch." The retreats include drug information education and peer counseling sessions. The counseling sessions are intended to serve as the basis for an ongoing peer support network among former participants, much as the group sessions in a treatment program may introduce addicts to 12-Step program peer support meetings. In addition to the counseling sessions, the retreat provided workshops on communication skills, refusal skills, goal-setting, problem-solving, and decision-making. At the end of the retreat, participants were encouraged to commit to individual short-term action plans in support of a healthy, drug-free life-style.

During the 14 weeks following the retreats, graduates of the program participated in four group counseling sessions designed to reinforce the material covered during the retreat experience. The group counseling sessions also provided opportunities to monitor the action plans and to help graduates develop longer-term goals and agendas.

Parent participation expected at the outset of the project did not materialize. The professional staff responsible for the implementation of the retreats consisted of a coordinator, two youth services specialists, and three teenage interns in the final stage of treatment at one of Amity's long-term addiction care facilities. All of the professional staff were well versed in substance abuse treatment technique, including group therapy and discussion sessions.

Outcome

Six months after the intervention, the participants were significantly more likely to report abstinence from "gateway" drug use compared with a group of similar risk status (see Figure 7.4). Teachers also reported positive changes in attitude and school performance. Working with adolescents identified as being at risk for drug use in the near future, the project demonstrated the potential of brief, intense interventions to reduce individual risk, at least during the short term.

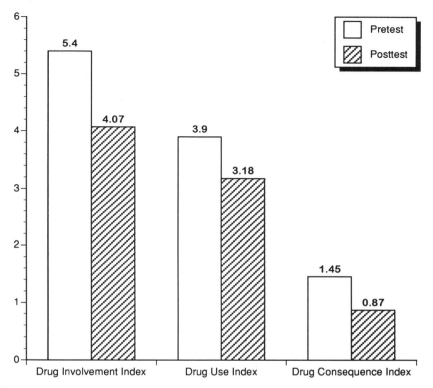

Figure 7.4. Peer support retreats: percentage of participants and control students reporting substance abuse during past 30 days.

─── **Contact**

Additional details on the peer support retreat program are found in Glider, Kressler, and McGrew (1991), an unpublished manuscript distributed by Amity, Inc., P.O. Box 32200, Tucson, AZ 85751-2200.

───────────────────────────── **PERSONAL GROWTH CLASS, WASHINGTON**

Personal Growth Class uses a specialized curriculum taught within a high school semester to intervene with older adolescents identified at high risk for drug use and other related outcomes.

Origin

The Personal Growth Class was developed by the Reconnecting At-Risk Youth Research Program at the University of Washington specifically to test the ability of public high schools to carry out an effective program for risk reduction among "problem" students. Research by Dr. Leona Eggert and her colleague, Liela J. Nicholas, associated teacher–student relationships, peer relationships, and the school environment with the progression of students from initial social problems to drug involvement, truancy, and school failure. The research team assumed that creating a social network among students identified at high risk for failure that provides mutual support for remaining in school can reduce both school drop-out rates and drug involvement.

Support for the program was provided by the National Institute on Drug Abuse and the State of Washington.

Implementation

The Personal Growth Class was established as an elective course that ran for the length of a 90-day semester. The overall program was administered by the school nurse. The nurse and four teacher/mentors received training from the course originators during a 3-day workshop, followed by weekly half-hour refresher sessions.

Topics covered in the Personal Growth Class included interpersonal communication, decision-making and goal-setting, stress management, study skills, career/work planning, and personal control over drug and alcohol use. Class enrollment was limited to a ratio of ten students to each teacher/mentor and to students identified by the high school authorities for any of the following:

- Previous history of dropding outs
- Below average grades
- High truancy rate
- Deficiencies in earned credit toward graduation
- Suspected drug use

A unique element of the curriculum is that specific skills training is introduced only after the absence of the skills is raised as an issue by the class participants. For example, rather than beginning training in effective decision-making at a predetermined point in the class syllabus, decision-making techniques were examined only after students initiate a discussion of the possibility that poor decision skills contribute to their personal problems. As explained by the creators of the Personal Growth Class,

An important intervention sequence was to first foster a group climate of expressed belonging and caring, then introduce skills training, positive reinforcement, monitoring behavioral changes, and celebrating goal achievements. (Moody & Eggert, 1992, p. 5)

————————————————————————————————— Outcome

A short-term evaluation of the Personal Growth Class was completed in 1990 (Eggert & Herting, 1991). Students in the Personal Growth Class documented a mean increase in grade point average from 1.5 to 1.8 at the end of 1 year and a similar increase in credits earned toward graduation. Matched controls documented sharp *decreases* in grades and credits earned during the study period.

After 10 months, students in the Personal Growth Class reported declines in the severity of drug-related problems and less spectacular declines in overall drug use, as measured by standardized index scales (see Figure 7.5). A comparison group of "normal" students who did not attend the Personal Growth Class tended to increase both their drug use and their experience of drug-related problems over the same time period. In addition, students in the Personal Growth Class tended to improve their grade point average significantly during the semester of the class; further improvement did not occur over the next 5 months (Eggert, Thompson, Herting, Nicholas, & Dicker, 1994).

————————————————————————————————— Contact

Detailed published sources on the Personal Growth Class include Eggert, Seyl, and Nicholas (1990) and Eggert *et al.* (1994). Dr. Leona L. Eggert can be contacted at CRN, Psychosocial Nursing Department, SC-76, University of Washington, Seattle, WA 98195.

**PROJECT HEALTHY ALTERNATIVES FOR LIFE'S
————————————————————————————— TRANSITIONS, NEBRASKA**

An alternative high school for students with behavioral problems received a program developed by substance abuse clinicians that sought to bring the content of outpatient drug abuse treatment into a classroom environment. The result was a time-limited intervention in a nonclinical setting that employed addiction specialists who used the behavior modification techniques found in clinical care.

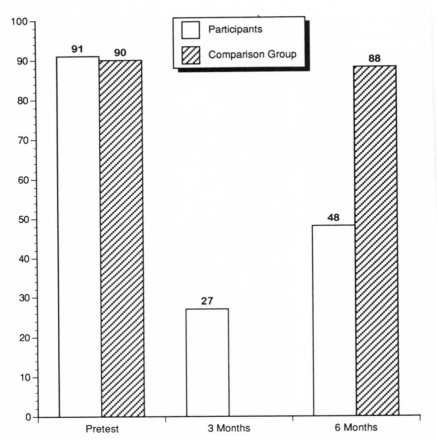

Figure 7.5. Personal Growth Class: mean change in selected drug use indices 10 months after participation. Source: Eggert and Herting (1991).

Origin

In 1987, Immanuel Mental Health Center of Omaha received a federal grant to develop and implement an early intervention curriculum for use in an alternative high school Approximately 60% of the students were identified as drug users.

Implementation

The curriculum for Project Healthy Alternatives for Life's Transitions (H.A.L.T.) includes education and group discussion and counseling related to drug use, self-esteem, assertiveness, problem solving, stress, and wellness. Part of the curriculum also discusses the roles that adolescents adopt to survive the stress of living in a dysfunctional family and provides suggestions on prevention of relapse to drug use. In effect, the H.A.L.T. curriculum compresses the education components of an outpatient addiction treatment program into 35 daily, 80-minute sessions.

As implemented in Omaha, the curriculum included speakers from a law enforcement agency to discuss legal issues of drug possession, and class trips to adolescent addiction treatment facilities. Students identified as potentially benefiting from self-help support groups were referred to meetings of Al-Anon, Nar-Anon, AA, and Narcotics Anonymous.

Ideal class size for Project H.A.L.T. was six to ten students; one-fourth of the student body of the alternative high school completed the course during its first year. It was assumed that participants would be referred by the school but in practice most students came to Project H.A.L.T. as self-referrals. Facilitators were recruited from the addiction treatment staff of the Mental Health Center.

Outcome

Teacher reports documented significant improvement in classroom behavior among former participants in the Project H.A.L.T. classes, measured by the number of disruptive incidents and reduced class and school absences. Self-esteem, as measured by a psychological testing instrument known as the Coopersmith battery, did not change (see discussion of self-esteem in Chapter 12).

Project H.A.L.T. permitted students to define their own short-term goals for drug, alcohol, and tobacco use. Few students tried to maintain complete abstinence during the first year and only one succeeded (see Figure 7.6). Nevertheless, given that the students already were assigned to an alternative school for behavioral problems, the small progress achieved by this intervention represents a lower-cost alternative to the addiction treatment that many of the students might otherwise eventually have needed.

Contact

Details on Project H.A.L.T. are derived from unpublished project documents submitted to the Center for Substance Abuse Prevention in 1989. The project curriculum is available for a nominal charge from the Immanuel Health Center, 6901 North 72nd Street, Omaha, NE 68122.

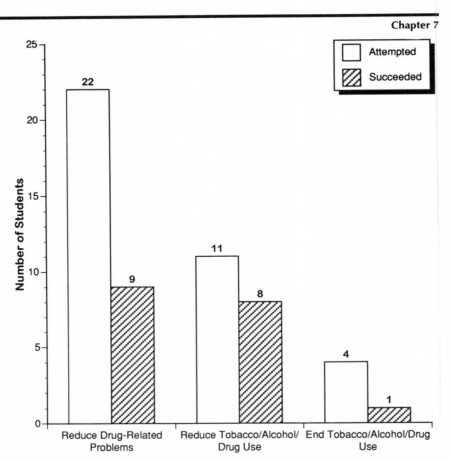

Figure 7.6. Project H.A.L.T.: number of students attempting and realizing personal goals.

RESIDENTIAL STUDENT ASSISTANCE PROGRAM, NEW YORK

Student Assistance Programs (SAPs), modeled after worksite Employee Assistance Programs (see Chapter 8), have a long history in public schools as an adjunct to the traditional school counselor. This initiative applied the approach to 13 to 19 year-olds assigned to Youth Homes and other residential facilities because of juvenile delinquency, severe emotional problems, and/or abuse or neglect.

Origin

The SAP model was refined in New York by the nonprofit Student Assistance Services Corporation during the early 1980s. Funding was provided by the State of New York, by the U.S. Department of Education, by the National Institute on Alcohol Abuse and Alcoholism, and by the Westchester County public schools. A CSAP grant supported adaptation of the model to residential facilities.

Implementation

The primary components of the SAP included the following:

- Professional alcohol and drug use assessments for all newly arriving residents
- Individual and group interpersonal counseling for residents who use alcohol or drugs, or who have an addicted parent
- Referral for treatment outside the residence for addicted youth
- Establishment of Adolescent Resident Task Forces that select drug abuse education activities for collaboration with SAP
- Institution of 12 Step meetings within the residences
- Ongoing professional training on substance abuse and children of alcoholic/addict concerns for residential facility staff
- Prevention education in the schools of the residential facilities, where permitted by school administrators, on the topics of tobacco, alcohol, and other drugs, family problems and pressures, and coping skills in problem-solving and stress management

Adolescent Task Forces develop activities on their own that benefit from access to SAP resources. These include smoking cessation classes, a Drug Free Club, peer counseling, and a poster contest.

A professional Student Assistance Counselor is assigned to each facility, with staff trainers and program evaluators operating from headquarters. Most counselors are former Child Protective Service or addiction treatment clinicians, selected for cultural match to the facility residents.

Program details vary widely among facilities. In some facilities, the counselor does not meet with youth during school hours; in others, the program is integrated with school-based efforts. Contact with family members is rare because the facilities tend to be far removed from the youths' previous homes.

Outcome

Placement in a residential facility deters access to alcohol and drugs. However, the residents visit their home and may work in the community, encountering situations where alcohol and drug use is possible. Over 2 years, opportunistic use of most drugs declined significantly (see Table 7.1), with the largest change

Table 7.1. New York SAP in Residential Facilities: Change in Percentage of Residents Reporting Current Drug Use following Program Implementation[a]

Substance	Percent of resident facility students reporting use in past 30 days (n=115)		
	1989	1990	Percentage change
Alcohol	38.9	34.4	−7.8
Marijuana	31.5	23.7	−24.7
Inhalants	10.4	9.4	−9.6
Hallucinogens	6.1	3.8	−37.7
Cocaine	6.1	6.9	+13.0
Crack cocaine	4.3	3.1	−27.9
Sedatives	4.3	0	−100.0
Tranquilizers	3.5	0	−100.0
Heroin	3.5	2.3	−34.3

[a]From Tobler, Kleinman, Morehouse, and Barkley (1991), p. 44.

in facilities where the SAP program collaborated with school-based efforts. Evaluators found a substantial effect of program participation on reduced quantity, frequency, and variety of drug use. According to Morehouse, Tobler, and Kleinman (1995), measured effect size of the SAP participation was 0.41, which suggests more extensive impact on behavior than most programs conducted among adolescents outside of a residential institution.

The project evaluation discovered that roughly 70% of youth entering residential facilities had received drug abuse prevention education in their home community—and were more likely to use drugs than the youth who had not experienced any drug abuse prevention education prior to entering the facility. This finding illustrates that many "general-purpose" prevention programs fail to affect the drug use behavior of "high-risk" youth.

Contacts

Details on SAP in residential facilities in New York State were derived from unpublished project documents submitted to CSAP in 1990–93 and from Morehouse *et al.* (1995). Additional information on the program can be obtained from the Student Assistance Services Corporation, 300 Farm Road, Ardsley, NY 10502.

The Office of the Safe and Drug-Free Schools Director in the Office of Superintendent of Public Instruction of the State of Washington independently completed a comprehensive review of the SAP approach in 1993.

SMART LEADERS (MULTISTATE)

The Boys and Girls Clubs of America, although perhaps less well known than the Boy Scouts and Girl Scouts, have been an important component of adolescent life in low-income areas for decades. During the 1980s, the clubs expanded beyond their traditional role of providing recreation and cultural programs by sponsoring the development of SMART Moves, a drug abuse prevention intervention for youth who enrolled in the Boys Clubs. SMART Moves initially consisted of Stay SMART, a program for younger adolescents. When the Boys Clubs found teenagers often requesting a follow-up program to help them cope with increased pressures to use alcohol or drugs as they entered high school, the Boys Clubs enlarged the program by developing SMART Leaders, an "advanced" drug abuse prevention initiative for older teenagers.

Origin

SMART Leaders was developed through a collaborative effort between Pennsylvania State University, Gilbert Botvin of Cornell University, and the Boys Clubs of America. The development of SMART Leaders became an opportunity to test whether the addition of booster sessions increases prevention effects of an initial intervention. Funding for an evaluation of SMART Leaders was provided by CSAP. At the same time, the Center also funded a study comparing indicators of substance abuse activity in public housing projects where Boys Clubs and SMART Moves were recently established with public housing where existing clubs did not implement SMART Moves and in other public housing where no Boys Clubs existed (Schinke *et al.*, 1991).

Implementation

Primary activities include five 90-minute sessions that reinforce drug education and resistance skills provided earlier in the Stay SMART program. In addition, the SMART Leaders I curriculum includes material on new skills for stress management, improving self-image, and assertiveness.

SMART Leaders II, provided to graduates of SMART Leaders I, consists of three modular sessions on alcohol, other drugs, and sexual activity, organized around videotape presentations. Unlike earlier components, SMART Leaders II emphasizes information rather than skill development.

The objective of the SMART Leaders program is to provide older boys with the knowledge and skills to serve as effective role models and peer advisors to the younger adolescents in the Boys Club program. Participants are Boys Club attendees identified as at risk for alcohol abuse or other drug use because of family, economic, or academic problems.

Outcome

An evaluation conducted by Pennsylvania State University compared drug use and drug-related attitudes among three groups:

- Youth who completed SMART Leaders and Stay SMART
- Youth who completed Stay SMART only
- Youth who did not receive any prevention services during the 27-month study period

Both the Stay SMART and SMART Leaders intervention groups reduced quantity and frequency of alcohol and tobacco use compared with youth who did not receive either program. They also showed more prosocial attitudes regarding teenage sexual activity. SMART Leaders participants averaged significantly lower levels of marijuana use than youth who did not receive booster sessions (see Figure 7.7). SMART Leaders demonstrated the importance of periodic reinforcement of prevention services in maintaining drug abstinence among high-risk youth.

The comparison of five Boys and Girls Clubs initiated in public housing projects with SMART Moves found a 13% reduction in juvenile criminal activity relative to public housing sites without Boys and Girls Clubs, measured by costs to repair youth vandalism and by police reports. The comparison also indicated a reduction in crack use and juvenile drug trafficking, although the measures for these outcomes may have reflected a certain amount of wishful thinking on the part of Boys and Girls Club personnel (Schinke *et al.*, 1991).

Contacts

Although these is an extensive literature on SMART Moves, the most comprehensive information is found in an unpublished final report submitted to CSAP in 1992 by the Institute for Policy Research and Evaluation of Pennsylvania State University. Information on the theory of SMART Moves and the multistate evaluation is available from the Institute for Policy Research, Pennsylvania State University, N253 Burrows Building, University Park, PA 16802. Additional information on SMART Moves is available from Marketing and Communications Services, Boys & Girls Clubs of America, 771 First Avenue, New York, NY 10017.

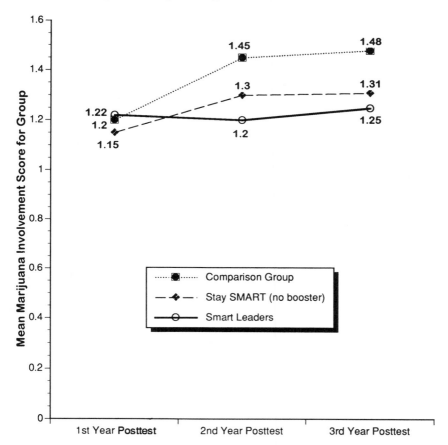

Figure 7.7. Stay SMART/SMART Leaders: mean change in participant marijuana involvement scores for selected groups.

GENERAL OBSERVATIONS

CSAP has focused support on intervention for so-called "high-risk" youth. This emphasis produced several programs that address multiple elements of the constellation of problems faced by youth at the highest risk for addiction. A few programs, such as CHOICE and the Personal Growth Class, center on classroom interventions. Others, such as the Peer Support Retreats, more closely resemble scaled-down addiction treatment programs.

Despite the significant differences in format, these successful interventions share important similarities in organization and staffing. First, the participating youth strongly influence the presentation of the material. This is clearly seen in the Personal Growth Class and the Resident Task Forces in the New York youth residences; it also is implicit in the CHOICE "self-help" groups and the group counseling of other programs. The key to success appears to be balancing the achievement of the planned goals of the curriculum with allowing participants to relate the learning to their own lives.

Another shared element is the focus on "life skills." All of the programs recognize the attraction of drug use as self-medication for teenagers with serious problems. Improving the ability to resolve problems through other means, such as stress reduction or decision-making, is probably more beneficial than giving them information about new drugs.

The importance of trained staff cannot be emphasized enough. In most of the successful programs, at least one individual on site is trained as a substance abuse counselor. The staff of the Everyday Theater Summer Program was well aware that the absence of a staff member with this training probably was damaging to the intervention. Good intentions and enthusiasm cannot substitute for a solid understanding of the needs of youth at risk. In addition, parents and other family members were either unavailable, as in the example of the Student Assistance Program, or chose not to participate.

All of the successful programs recognized that adolescents in trouble are still adolescents. Program content often was structured around role-playing and other games, dramatic exercises, field trips, and other elements that appeal to children. These were not recreational activities for the sake of recreation; rather, this was "fun" with a serious instructional or skill-building function in mind. The objective was to make behavior change enjoyable without losing sight of the specific tasks that the program designers want to accomplish to reduce the risk for future addiction.

Finally, as with programs designed to help families in trouble, the most successful examples of preventive initiatives designed for adolescents at greatest risk for drug involvement often concentrate resources on identifying the youth who can use help. This was not a problem in the shelter for homeless youth in New Haven, the alternative high school in Omaha, or the youth residences in New York; it was, however, important for programs that operated within main-stream institutions. As noted by Leona Eggert and her colleagues,

> The point is that programs aimed at all students may not be needed by some and, more importantly, may be insufficient for others. Targeting extensive, high-dosage interventions at only identified high-risk youth is more economical and has a greater potential for effectiveness with those who need it. (Eggert *et al.*, 1994, p. 205)

Problem: Preventing Substance Abuse among Employees and Retirees

People often view substance abuse as a teenage problem because it usually begins with youthful experimentation in alcohol and tobacco. They may forget that many people probably first try illegal drugs as adults. Figure 8.1 shows that half of all adults who ever used marijuana tried it for the first time during or after their late teen years. In addition, most teenagers classified as substance abusers fall into that category because they are using legal drugs before the minimum purchase age; as soon as they reach their 21st birthday, they technically stop being abusers. The same cannot be said for young adults who become involved in drug use.

Of approximately 24 million Americans who used an illegal drug during the past year, a majority are over 25 years old. Older Americans also are much more likely than youth to drink alcoholic beverages every week; for example, over one-third of American men over 35 consume at least one drink per week, compared with roughly 30% of men between the ages of 18 and 25 and only 6% of teenage boys (see Figure 8.2, page 115).

From the above, it is obvious that serious prevention of alcohol- and drug-related problems must invest at least some resources in prevention for populations beyond secondary school. At the least, the absence of adult prevention contributes to health problems among the elderly, to drug-related incidents at work, and to a new generation of drug-abusing parents who may pass their substance abuse habits on to their children.

It is difficult to initiate substance abuse prevention for adults. There is little consensus about the extent to which prevention of substance abuse among adults should be left up to the individual or should be at least in part a community responsibility. Some policymakers who support publicly funded prevention efforts for youth believe that adult drug use should be deterred by criminal justice

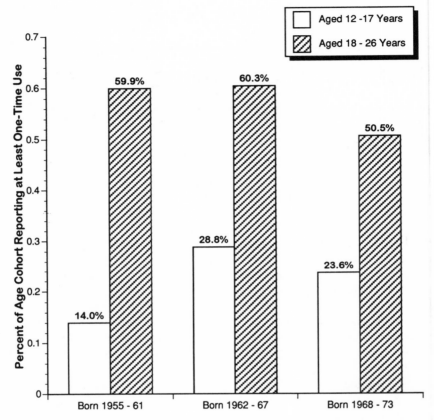

Figure 8.1. Lifetime experience with marijuana use: three birth cohorts during adolescence and young adulthood. Data derived from National Household Surveys on Drug Use, 1972–1991.

sanctions. In effect, they argue that society should teach children to avoid drugs but should punish them if they haven't learned the lesson as adults. Charitable groups soliciting funds for prevention efforts recognize that a 23-year-old working man or woman living alone, smoking tobacco, and drinking alcoholic beverages is an unattractive drug abuse "poster child" to would-be donors.

Even the healthcare system has an ambivalent attitude toward substance abuse prevention among adults. Insurers have been generous contributors to community efforts to curb youth substance abuse. Since passage of the Drug-Free Workplace Act of 1988, however, many insurers have taken the position that employers, rather than the healthcare system, should respond to adult drug

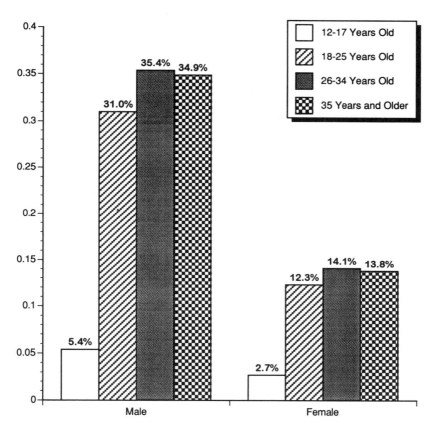

Figure 8.2. Percentage of age groups reporting weekly consumption of alcoholic beverages, 1991. Data derived from National Household Surveys on Drug Use, 1972–1991.

use with preemployment drug screening and swift, certain dismissal from employment for drug possession. Some healthcare carriers have urged extending antidrug policies to exclude tobacco users and alcohol abusers from employment—and from health insurance coverage.

BARRIERS TO ADULT PREVENTION

When the community wants to work with adults and earmarks funds for this purpose, effective substance abuse prevention beyond school-age populations

often remains an elusive goal. Three major issues complicate preventive interventions for adults:

- Science has not yet conclusively explained why people begin to use
  illegal drugs or abuse alcohol as adults.
- Adults are more difficult than youth to reach with effective prevention
  messages.
- Research has not focused on prevention techniques that are effective
  among adults.

Regarding the first issue, the problem is not that scientists lack theories for
late-onset use of illegal drugs or alcoholism but rather that there is little support
for research to test these theories. We know, for example, that when people leave
a supervised home environment, they suddenly have greater opportunity to
indulge in previously forbidden behavior including drug abuse. They may move
from an abstinent environment to one in which drug use or heavy drinking is
encouraged, or to a community where they believe that "everyone else is using"
(Perkins, 1994). College students pledging a fraternity or military recruits on
leave after completing basic training, for example, may find themselves in
situations where they assume that staying sober is considered abnormal. What
we don't know is whether this is a major route to adult substance abuse problems
or merely part of a process of developing problems that begins earlier in life.

Sociologists believe that similar influences may explain why some immigrants develop substance abuse problems after they arrive in the United States.
Young arrivals to this country may interpret the apparent freedom to drink
alcoholic beverages and use drugs to be part of the U.S. experience which they
want to adopt. Alternatively, the drinking or drug use patterns that are considered
normal in some countries may be defined as abuse in the United States. For
example, outdoor social beer drinking among unmarried men is an evening
tradition in Mexico but often is viewed as unacceptable behavior in this country
(e.g., see Caetano & Medina-Mora, 1990) while the coca leaf tea viewed as a
staple in the mountains of Bolivia and Colombia raises the spectre of cocaine
abuse in the United States.

Unwholesome expression of freedom and independence is only one possible mechanism for adult onset of substance abuse. Other sources include

- Dependence as a by-product of the aging process, when the body no
  longer can tolerate the amount of alcohol or a medication dosage that
  previously could be harmlessly consumed (Atkinson, Tolson, & Turner,
  1990)
- Efforts to self-medicate a mental health problem

■ Unexpected pressures and stress, including loss of a spouse or the sudden increase in free time that comes with retirement (e.g., see references in Minnis, 1990)

The very limited research available has not produced credible numbers indicating which of these are important and which are minor causes of late-onset problems. The rate of substance abuse among the elderly is particularly controversial, with some estimates suggesting widespread development of "hidden" substance abuse problems following retirement, while clinical data suggest that the only widespread geriatric substance abuse problem may be accidental overdose of prescription medication. Sidney Schnoll, M.D., of Virginia Commonwealth University Medical Center, is one of the most active supporters of preventive interventions targeted among older potential substance abusers, but he notes that there has been strong resistance to collection of baseline data among the elderly (conversation with Dr. Schnoll at the Second National NIDA Conference on Drug Abuse Research and Practice, Washington, DC, July 16, 1993).

Assuming that we understood the process through which adults develop substance abuse problems, there are few methods to inexpensively identify adults in need of help and to provide effective intervention. The Partnership for a Drug-Free America has tried to blanket the broadcast media with anti-drug abuse messages that may reinforce existing attitudes and contribute to antidrug opinions. However, the available evidence suggests that the Partnership's 30-second television spots do not actually change individual behavior. In earlier decades, there was a reasonable possibility of reaching the majority of young men with powerful prevention messages during military service, but the advent of the all-volunteer army eliminated this cost-effective approach.

Today, the most effective adult prevention programs focus their energy on a few key sites rather than trying to blanket a community with prevention messages. The efforts discussed here are limited to examples of the few worksite and community workshop prevention programs that collected outcome data. Chapter 2 cited interventions for pregnant women at health clinics and Chapter 9 includes campus and responsible beverage service programs.

AETNA HAI MANAGED BEHAVIORAL HEALTH, UTAH

As noted earlier, employees receiving workplace health benefits increasingly are covered under managed care programs. Managed care aggressively controls access and costs for medical services. The Human Affairs International (HAI) subsidiary of Aetna Life Insurance Company is a provider of mental health managed care and employee assistance programs that has found that investing in preventive worksite interventions is more effective and less costly than traditional means of identifying and treating employees with alcohol abuse, drug use, and mental health problems.

Origin

Some programs that claim to be "managed care" providers focus on serving as a gatekeeper to medical services. This type of program usually consists of a telephone-based screening and review conducted by mental health professionals to determine what kind of care an employee may need.

In 1989, Aetna HAI offered corporate insurance purchasers a choice between this minimalist approach to cost reduction and a more aggressive Managed Behavioral Health (MBH) program. The following year, Aetna compared cost and clinical service utilization for 41,400 employees covered by MBH with costs and services used by 173,750 employees covered by Aetna HAI's traditional managed care.

Implementation

MBH is a comprehensive approach emphasizing prevention of employee mental health problems before they require extensive clinical care. Worksites under MBH receive the services of an employee assistance program (EAP) that includes education and in-person counseling. The EAP professionals offer advice and referral to self-help support groups, and focus on underlying life stresses that may contribute to substance abuse and mental health problems. Additional cost control is accomplished through networks of preferred providers and case management.

Outcome

After 27 months of monitoring costs, and controlling for differences in the demography of employees under the two approaches, Aetna HAI concluded that MBH saved 19.8% on net mental health and addiction treatment costs over traditional managed care. Specifically,

- Worksites covered by MBH saved an annual average of $54 per employee in addiction and mental health care expenses compared with a limited gatekeeper approach.
- Worksites covered by MBH saved an annual average of $190 per employee in total health costs.

■ Among employees eventually referred to inpatient addiction treatment, average length of stay for the MBH patients was 20 days compared with 23.7 days for patients from the traditional managed care system.

Employees who received the interventions of MBH were thus less likely to need costly mental health and addiction care or other healthcare, and averaged less inpatient treatment than employees who were covered by traditional managed care.

Contact

Data on the evaluation of the Aetna program appeared in a release issued by Aetna Life Insurance Company in July, 1992. Additional information is available from Phil Quigley, Product Manager, Managed Behavioral Health, P.O. Box 57986, Salt Lake City, UT 84157-0986.

LEVI-STRAUSS WORKSITE POLICY CHANGES, TENNESSEE

The initial concept of an EAP was to identify employees with an alcohol or other drug-related problem and refer them to counseling, treatment, or self-help programs. This reactive approach to substance abuse problems is being replaced in many companies by an EAP that promotes sober, healthy life-styles and identifies company policies and customs that encourage abuse. The changes implemented in the Levi Strauss garment manufacturing firm, as a result of experience at one plant in Tennessee, are typical of this trend.

Origin

An on-site EAP was instituted at a rural Levi Strauss facility in response to a management request for a program to address the many alcohol, drug, and social issues plaguing the work force. Over a period of 6 years, the EAP acted as a catalyst for changing corporate policy with a general objective of cost containment for medical and related expenses.

Implementation

The EAP achieved an annual 10% utilization rate, with an increase of 278% between 1990 and 1993. Preemployment drug tests and a general health promotion approach were implemented. Other policy reforms included the elimination of management-sanctioned use of alcohol as part of workplace sales celebrations. The company's benefit department also developed managed care guidelines governing employee treatment for drug abuse.

Outcome

Since instituting the program, the Levi Strauss plant sales force has experienced dramatic declines in alcohol use. In addition, the plant documented declining use of mental health and other healthcare benefits, with cost savings accruing to the company. The EAP and related policy changes have since been adopted in other Levi Strauss facilities throughout the United States and in several foreign countries.

Contact

Information on this program was presented to an expert panel on worksite substance abuse prevention convened by the Center for Substance Abuse Prevention in February, 1995. The presenter was Dr. Margaret Kraemer, EAP of Levi Strauss & Company, P.O. Box 15906, Knoxville, TN 37901.

LOS ANGELES WATER AND POWER SUPERVISORY TRAINING PROGRAM, CALIFORNIA

Most adults who have substance abuse issues may never require clinical treatment. Instead, they may need only a brief intervention to become aware of the issue and of self-care approaches that can correct the problem. This is the philosophy behind the National Institute of Alcohol Abuse and Alcoholism campaign to instruct primary care physicians in the use of tools to help patients with alcohol-related problems (National Institute on Alcohol Abuse and Alcoholism, 1995). It also justifies the role of worksite EAPs as a combined intervention and referral service for workers with substance abuse problems.

AlthoughEAPs provide health education for worksites, they usually cannot offer personal intervention to every employee. The Department of Water and Power of Los Angeles experimented with training supervisors to better focus the prevention, intervention, and treatment services of the EAP on those workers who need professional help.

Origin

An annual review of the EAP of the Los Angeles City Department of Water and Power discovered significant outcome differences between employees who referred themselves to the EAP for alcohol-related problems and employees referred to the EAP by a supervisor. The voluntary referrals *increased* their average number of medical absences following self-referral to the alcohol intervention program, from 96.8 hours per year to 144.8 hours per year. In contrast, employees who were referred to alcohol intervention by their supervisors *reduced* their average use of medical leave from 117.4 hours per year to 78.4 hours per year. In effect, employees identified and referred for alcohol problems by their supervisor tended to be more troubled than the self-referred employees but also were more likely to eventually return to the worksite's average rate for frequency of employee absence.

The directors of the EAP decided that these results argued strongly for increasing the rate of supervisor referral of employees for alcohol-related problems. Their program was designed to make supervisors more effective allies of the EAP by training them to be more aggressive in making referrals for serious cases.

Implementation

The process of improving the supervisor referral consisted of two phases. The first phase was clarifying the requirements for a formal supervisory referral. Although the EAP had long distinguished between formal and informal referrals, the program had never spelled out in clear terms the process for a formal referral. Written guidelines and a short policy statement were issued before supervisors were trained, and a follow-up form was created to give supervisors a tool to monitor the performance of employees after an intervention for substance abuse-related problems.

The second phase of the program consisted of training supervisors to use the new guidelines and follow-up form effectively. Departmentwide management training included the detailed discussion of the referral procedures, emphasizing the appropriateness of making mandatory referrals. After the training, medical personnel attached to the department were instructed in how to encourage supervisors on an ongoing basis to make formal referrals.

Outcome

The new policy statement and supervisor training resulted in a dramatic increase in the percentage of the EAP intervention caseload from formal supervisor referral (see Figure 8.3). Based on earlier data, the department estimated that supervisor training saved approximately $250,000 in absenteeism costs during its first year of operation.

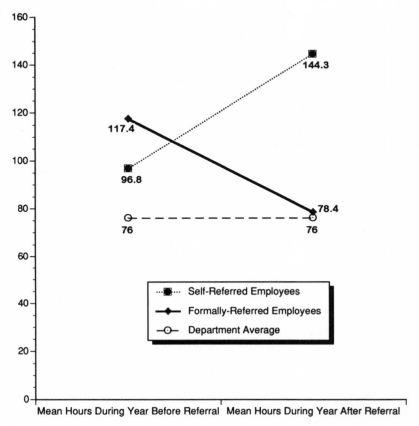

Figure 8.3. Los Angeles Water and Power Department: absenteeism among employees before and after alcohol-problem referral.

Contact

Data on the Los Angeles City Water and Power program was derived from Amaral and Cross's *Cost-Benefits of Supervisory Referrals*, an unpublished paper prepared for the 1988 Annual Conference of the Employee Assistance Program Association of Los Angeles. Additional information is available from Susan Cross, Director, Employee Assistance Program, Department of Water and Power, City of Los Angeles, 717 West Temple Street, Los Angeles, CA 90012.

————————— MENTAL HEALTH AND AGING WORKSHOPS, OREGON

Mental health problems, including substance abuse, among older adults are strongly linked to physical and social functioning. The ability to stay sober, alert, and involved in the community can mean the difference between independent living and custodial care for an elderly American. Oregon State University developed a community education program designed to alert older people and caregivers to geriatric substance abuse and other mental health problems. Alcohol abuse, for example, is estimated to occur among as many as 10% of the unmarried population over 65 years old. It often is clinically ignored because physicians assume that memory lapse, inappropriate drowsiness, and other alcohol-related symptoms are the result of old age. In fact, a significant portion of geriatric substance abuse consists of drinking alcoholic beverages while taking medication for chronic age-related conditions (Minnis, 1990). Intervention can identify issues in time to prevent them from becoming serious problems.

—————————————————————————————————— **Origin**

Two statewide task forces in 1986 reported that lack of information on alcoholism, drug abuse, and mental illness among senior citizens frequently delayed identification of developing problems. The task forces identified three priority areas

- Alcohol and drug use, abuse, and dependence among older Americans
- Coping with the loss of spouse, health, job, friends, and so on
- Mental and emotional problems specific to aging

The task forces also wanted an educational effort to reduce the stigma associated with older people receiving mental health and substance abuse services. The same items were identified in a needs assessment survey of attendees at Oregon State University (OSU) Extension programs on aging during 1984–86.

In response to these needs, the OSU Extension Service developed three model workshops to raise awareness and educate senior citizens, family members, and community caregivers. OSU also promoted the dissemination of the workshops in Oregon. Funding was provided by the state, by the U.S. Administration on Aging, and indirectly by the U.S. Department of Agriculture through its support for state extension services.

—————————————————————————————————— **Implementation**

The three workshops developed by OSU are

- *Winter Comforts,* focused on alcohol problems

■ *The Final Course* on potentially suicidal depression
■ *The Second Story*, a workshop on loss

The core of each workshop is a 15- to 20-minute slide-and-sound media program that humanizes the topic by illustrating the problems of one older person and her family. For *Winter Comforts*, the slide-and-sound presentation focuses on a 72-year-old woman who had developed a late-onset alcohol problem.

The other elements of the workshop package are

■ Instructions for organizing the workshop
■ Step-by-step workshop guide, including a script of the media presentation and overhead transparencies
■ Publicity materials
■ Skill-building activities for workshop participants, including worksheets and handouts
■ Instructions on how to locate local resources

The initial development of the workshop materials was followed by full-day training sessions for individuals who were likely to present the programs in their home communities. The training sessions were organized by county agricultural extension agents, who worked with county health offices, area agencies on aging, and housing and care facilities for the elderly. Eventually 2000 future workshop presenters received the training and workshop package.

Outcome

Evaluations of each of the three workshop programs were conducted among participants in the statewide workshop facilitator training and among participants in the community workshops.

A comparison of pretest and posttest questionnaires found that the participants as a group displayed significant improvement in the ability to accurately answer questions related to alcohol problems and mental health issues among older Americans. On a ten-item alcohol knowledge questionnaire, for example, participants' mean score rose from 7.8 to 8.7 correct answers, while the average score for nonparticipants *fell* from 7.1 to 6.6.

The program also influenced behavioral intention toward people who may have alcohol problems. By the posttest, workshop participants were significantly more likely than nonparticipants to believe they will actively intervene or seek help for prevention of further alcohol problems among senior citizens in the community (see Figure 8.4).

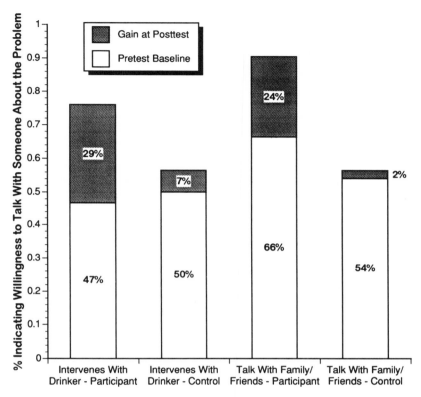

Figure 8.4. Oregon Mental Health and Aging Workshops: "very likely"/"definitely would" answers on behavioral intent in response to elderly drinking problem.

─── **Contact**

The Oregon Mental Health and Aging Workshops were described in an unpublished project report submitted by Oregon State University to the U.S. Administration on Aging in August, 1991. Copies of the workshop package are available at cost from Extension Home Economics, Milam Hall 161, Oregon State University, Corvallis, OR 97331-5106. A videotape version of the slide-and-sound program also is available for individual or small group use.

─── **GENERAL OBSERVATIONS**

Very few substance abuse prevention programs for adults generate data that could prove or disprove their effectiveness. Most public sector research on reducing adult drug use has been devoted to the cost-benefit of addiction treatment and criminal justice penalties. No study directly compares the effectiveness of preventive interventions to either of the other two approaches in driving adult drug use from the community. Of course, no community would abandon either treatment or law enforcement and rely solely on prevention in responding to adult drug use; however, the lack of such comparative data reinforces the willingness of some communities to ignore prevention as an approach suitable for adults. In 1995, for example, Congress voted to virtually eliminate all federal funding for worksite substance abuse prevention demonstration projects.

Without a strong, consistent public commitment to substance abuse prevention for adults, most efforts targeted at individuals over high school age have been organized and funded by the private sector, including employers, insurers, and medical care providers. Few privately funded efforts, however, collect adequate data on the specific interventions that work. The examples of the Levi Strauss employee assistance program and the Aetna HAI Managed Behavioral Health program are atypical because they collected data beyond the subjective opinions of workers and supervisors. However, like many other private sector programs, they documented that the entire package of interventions appeared to have had an impact on adult populations and do not offer insights into which components of the package were essential and which were ineffective in producing the results.

The following chapter, focusing specifically on community responses to adult alcohol abuse, provides further evidence that preventive interventions can be effective among older Americans. In fact, as a society, the United States has had greater success in reducing adult alcohol abuse and tobacco use than in reducing the incidence of many adolescent substance abuse problems. Scientists, however, have not had access to the data that would explain how this success among adults was achieved. Perhaps the cost-consciousness of the managed care environment will extend to prevention of adult alcohol and drug abuse, producing studies with more useful designs and greater rigor to explain what works.

9

Problem: Reducing the Costs of Alcohol Use

In 1987, Secretary of Health and Human Services Otis Bowen proclaimed "alcohol is a drug" and ordered his department to refer to "alcohol and other drug abuse" in place of "substance abuse." These actions were hailed by many preventionists as a victory in treating alcohol as part of the national drug problem. Others argued that describing alcohol as a "drug" ignores important differences between alcohol and other abused substances.

Alcohol is not viewed by most of the public as belonging to the same category as cocaine and heroin. Unlike other drugs, alcoholic beverages are legal and socially acceptable. They are a traditional part of the religious practices, social life, and diet of millions of Americans. Beverage advertising and sales are essential to the profits of hundreds of legitimate businesses; alcohol-related revenue is critical to the government budgets of several states. Finally, clinical evidence suggests that limited alcohol consumption is either physically harmless or beneficial for most people; dietary guidelines issued by the U.S. Department of Health and Human Services in 1996 recommend a very limited consumption of alcohol as a possible protective factor against certain types of heart and blood diseases.

In effect, while it may be technically accurate to refer to alcohol as a drug, the role of alcoholic beverages in human affairs and health since the dawn of recorded history places alcohol in a special niche in the substance abuse field. This may have been one of the reasons why the U.S. Department of Health and Human Services quietly reversed Secretary Bowen's order in 1996, stating that "substance abuse" is again the preferred term to "alcohol and other drug abuse."

The unique status of alcoholic beverages make prevention of alcohol abuse significantly more complex than prevention of illegal drug abuse. The goal usually is to permit legal access to alcoholic beverages while reducing the cost of misuse of alcohol. In other words, society does not try to prevent alcohol consumption but rather to prevent alcohol consumption at the wrong time, by the wrong people, in the wrong amounts.

BEHIND THE MYTH OF AN ALCOHOLIC SOCIETY ━━━━━━

Many prevention advocates describe the United States as an "alcoholic society." They suggest that alcohol is pervasive in our culture, with children indoctrinated at any early age into drinking behavior. At the same time, alcohol generates higher medical costs than all illegal drugs combined (mostly the result of alcohol-related traffic injuries). Preventionists also point out that alcohol use is associated with sexual assault, child and spouse abuse, other drug use, and dozens of social ills.

Other facts, however, undermine the indictment that United States today has a societal drinking problem:

- Americans formerly drank much more. The expense accounts of the Founding Fathers generally reveal daily consumption of awesome amounts of wine, rum, brandy, and alcoholic punch. Documented per capita purchase of alcoholic beverages other than beer and wine peaked in 1977 at about one-third above current consumption.
- Roughly half of all Americans who use alcoholic beverages average fewer than four drinks per week.
- Most Americans who use alcoholic beverages never "graduate" to other drugs and experience no serious problems from alcohol use.
- The United States has among the highest rates of alcohol abstinence of any wealthy country, ranging from 32% among adult males nationally to 63% among adult women in the South (Williams & DeBakey, 1992).

This last statistic is significant because it highlights the extent to which alcohol consumption varies by region. For example, more than 60% of all adults in Georgia abstain completely from alcohol, but the average drinker in that state consumes the equivalent of a fifth of vodka per week. In contrast, as shown in Figure 9.1, Connecticut has one of the lowest abstinence rates in the country but mean consumption is about half that of Peach State drinkers (Williams, Stinson, Brooks, Clem, & Noble, 1991). Nationally about 10% of adults consume half of the alcohol sold—and are believed responsible for most alcohol-related problems.

Alcoholics probably constitute a large subset of frequent drinkers. However, alcohol dependence often is difficult to distinguish from "normal" heavy drinking. Many people who drink heavily during their youth gradually reduce intake without ever experiencing withdrawal. Children of alcoholics are more likely than average to develop alcohol dependence, but the majority of even this population never develop alcoholism. In effect, it isn't practical to either predict alcohol dependence or to prevent it without restricting access to the drug.

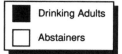

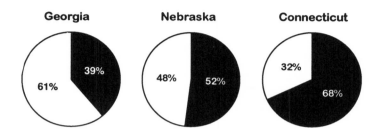

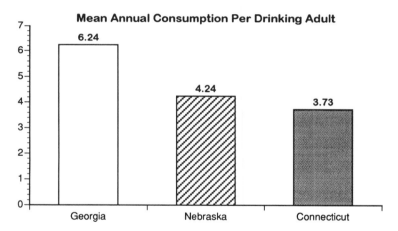

Figure 9.1. Estimated apparent per capita annual alcohol consumption in gallons for adults in three states. Source: G. D. Williams, E. S. Stinson, S. D. Brooks, D. Clem, and J. Noble. (1991). *Apparent per capita alcohol consumption: National, state, and regional trends, 1977–1989* [NIAAA Surveillance Report No. 20, DHHS Publication No. (ADM)281–89–0001]. Washington, DC: Superintendent of Documents.

A viable alternative to attempting to reduce alcohol dependence is to target prevention to one or more of four abusive behaviors:

■ Operating a vehicle or other equipment under the influence of alcohol

- Underage drinking (in states where there is a minimum age for consumption in addition to the national minimum age of 21 years for purchase of alcoholic beverages)
- Recurring intoxication, particularly if linked to violence, sexual misconduct, or poor work performance
- Frequent consumption and consumption at inappropriate times

Each solution described in this chapter addresses at least one of these behaviors. At the same time, designers of alcohol problem interventions often suggest that their efforts help reduce the incidence of alcohol dependence. If true, this would be a valuable side benefit from prevention aimed at more easily identifiable problems.

ALCOHOL, DRUGS, DRIVING, AND YOU, COLORADO

Automobile crashes are the leading cause of death among young adults in the United States. Although most fatal crashes do *not* involve a drinking or drug-impaired driver, teenagers and young adults remain about twice as likely as other Americans to be victims of an alcohol-related traffic incident. Even communities that appear tolerant of teenage drinking are likely to support a high school intervention program that focuses specifically on alcohol-impaired driving and managed healthcare companies recognize that this is one substance abuse problem area that directly affects their financial bottom line. Alcohol, Drugs, Driving, and You (ADDY) is a comprehensive package that meets the need for this type of program using a school-based curriculum.

Origin

ADDY was developed by The Prevention Center, a nonprofit corporation in Boulder, Colorado. Emphasizing the need to change norms away from risk-taking while driving, ADDY is designed to be used in either tenth-grade health or driver education classes. In 1984, the program was extensively field-tested in secondary schools in Colorado (see Camilli & Brennan, 1984), and then revised. During the next 5 years, use of ADDY spread throughout the United States.

Implementation

ADDY includes lessons on the effects of alcohol and drugs on driving, legal consequences, decision making skills, and techniques to resist peer influence on risk-taking. The curriculum can be taught in five classroom sessions or can require as many as 15, depending on the number of suggested activities used by the students. Classroom teachers are trained to deliver ADDY through an instructional video provided by The Prevention Center. Other elements of the ADDY package are an extensive teacher manual, a guide to involving the tenth-grade students in planning community and school awareness events, a parent guide, and a media kit.

Outcome

The national version of the ADDY curriculum was evaluated by comparing responses of program participants with those of controls in schools that did not participate in ADDY. The comparison found significant benefits for knowledge gains and for avoidance of riding with alcohol- or drug-impaired drivers. The desired attitude changes were more pronounced among female than male participants (Fleming & Davis, 1987).

Contact

Descriptions and evaluations of ADDY are found in Camilli and Brennan (1984) and Fleming and Davis (1987). Additional information is available from Lisa Thompson, Colorado Resource Prevention Center, 7525 West 10th Avenue, Lakewood, CO 80215-5141.

ALCOHOLIC BEVERAGE SERVER INTERVENTION (MULTISTATE)

Several training programs for beverage server personnel have been found to reduce alcohol abuse. Such training changes the environment from one in which each drinker is solely responsible for limiting his consumption to one in which the server and the establishment share an interest in limiting consumption.

Origin

Server intervention, or responsible beverage service, is an update and codification of policies suggested by Jim Peters and James F. Mosher for states where beverage servers are held legally liable for harm inflicted by their drunken patrons. Responsible beverage service programs represent a response to the threat of such "dram shop liability" litigation against bar owners and to the discovery that nearly a third of alcohol-related accidents are caused by drivers leaving bars and restaurants (see Fell, 1988).

Implementation

Responsible beverage service or server intervention programs usually consist of the following three elements:

- Development of a clearly stated responsible beverage service policy for retail outlets
- Training servers to meet the requirements of the policy, including checking identification to prevent underage drinking, offering food and nonalcoholic beverages, and stopping service when appropriate
- Training servers in specific intervention techniques and skills, including cues to identify patrons at risk of severe alcohol-related consequences

Communities and insurance companies have been known to encourage implementation of responsible beverage service in several ways, including making adoption of responsible beverage service a precondition for beverage license issuance or renewal, and using documentation of responsible beverage service as a trigger for reduction in insurance premiums. Merely increasing the penalties for violation of dram shop liability laws was linked to elimination of low-price promotions and refusal of service to intoxicated patrons. However, changes in dram shop liability alone do not seem to be enough to motivate bar owners and restauranteurs to implement formal server intervention training or checks for patron age (Holder *et al.*, 1993).

Outcomes

Government, the beverage industry, and the research community have collaborated on several relatively rigorous evaluations of the effects of this prevention approach. Among the dozens of evaluations of the impact of server interventions, three studies stand out as both rigorous and convincing. These three studies are the Gator Gardens evaluation and the Training for Intervention Procedures by Servers (TIPS) evaluation, funded by the National Institute on Alcohol Abuse and Alcoholism (NIAAA), and a national multisite evaluation conducted by the National Highway Transportation Safety Administration (NHTSA).

The Gator Gardens Server Intervention Program examined the effects of server training at an enlisted men's club on a large naval base. Most club patrons were men between the ages of 18 and 25 (Navy policy then permitted all personnel on base to buy beer in spite of civilian drinking age laws). During the 2 months after server training, evaluators noted significant reductions in the hourly rate of consumption of alcoholic beverages and in the percentage of patrons consuming drink sizes that normally produce intoxication (see Figure

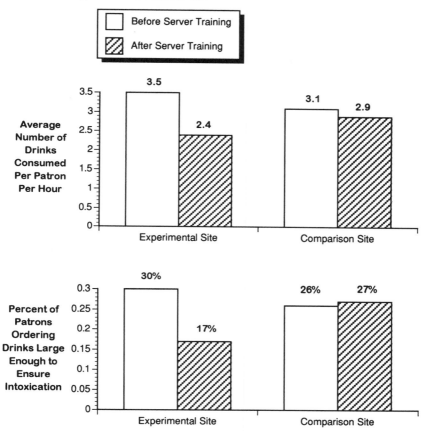

Figure 9.2. Server intervention at Gator Gardens: pretest/posttest differences in patron behavior.

9.2). Per capita consumption did not change as a result of a slight mean increase among light drinkers. Such changes were absent in a nearby club with untrained servers (Saltz, 1987).

The evaluation of TIPS, like Gator Gardens, was another relatively early systematic study of the impact of server intervention. TIPS was provided to half of the servers in two establishments in southwestern Virginia. Comparisons were made with the behavior of untrained server personnel at the same locations. Trained servers conducted more interventions than untrained servers to reduce consumption. Patrons of trained servers averaged lower blood alcohol concentration on leaving the establishment than patrons served by untrained staff. The TIPS evaluation also found, surprisingly, that trained servers averaged higher income from tips than untrained servers. The researchers believed that the increased contact with patrons encouraged by server intervention training resulted in a more favorable view of the servers, even when the servers were trying to encourage patrons to slow down on their alcohol consumption (Russ & Geller, 1987).

The most ambitious evaluation of server intervention was sponsored by NHTSA. It included more than 100 outlets in eight states. Evaluators observed that trained servers were significantly more likely than untrained servers to provide an intervention to discourage consumption by drunken patrons. However, the servers were not more likely to increase the number of occasions on which they denied drinks to intoxicated patrons. The evaluators concluded that responsible beverage policies affect server behavior but may not alter patron behavior enough to prevent most alcohol-impaired driving (see Figure 9.3). In

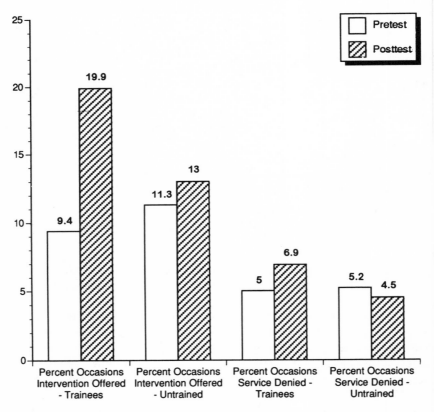

Figure 9.3. NHTSA Responsible Alcohol Service Project: changes in server intervention.

addition, the effectiveness of server intervention appeared to be affected by the volume of business and the typical clientele (such as blue-collar versus white-collar) at each location (McKnight, 1991).

A final concern about responsible beverage service is that server training effects tend to be short-lived because of rapid turnover among bar and restaurant employees. Server intervention training must be conducted repeatedly and policies must be reinforced with incentives to sustain the desired effects.

Contact

Several perspectives on server intervention were published in a special 1985 issue of *Alcohol Health & Research World*; a more recent review of the literature is Saltz (1989). Consultants specializing in responsible beverage programs include Health Communications, Inc., 1101 Wilson Boulevard., Suite 1700, Arlington, VA 22209, which provides TIPS training; the Business Council for Alcohol Education, P.O. Box 3406, Phoenix, AZ 85030; and the National Licensed Beverage Association, 4214 King Street, Alexandria, VA 22314. In California, the Responsible Beverage Service Coalition of Napa County offers a training program designed to meet the needs of regions where wine tasting is a popular tourist attraction; the Coalition is located at Suite H, 1561 Third Street, Napa, CA 94559.[1]

COMMUNITY ALCOHOL ABUSE AND INJURY PREVENTION PROJECT, RHODE ISLAND

CAAIPP demonstrated that changing the behavior of individuals involved in alcohol policy formulation and enforcement can reduce the number of severe alcohol-related problems.

Origin

The Rhode Island CAAIPP began in 1984 as a partnership between the NIAAA, the Rhode Island Department of Health, and the U.S. Centers for Disease Control and Prevention. Its purpose was to determine whether changing the community environment alone can reduce alcohol-related problems, including injuries.

----

[1] References provided by Mindy K. Stein, Administrator, Licensed Beverage Information Council.

Implementation

The 5-year project emphasized server training in responsible service of alcoholic beverages among all bars and restaurants in the community of Woonsocket and police training and improvement in enforcement of alcohol-related laws. In addition, CAAIPP relied on community mobilization and publicity, including enlisting civic and political leaders in support of the program.

Outcome

Woonsocket police met the goal of identifying more arrests other than driving under the influence cases as alcohol-related. Beverage servers in Woonsocket practiced more frequent interventions to reduce potential problems among their drinking patrons. Neither change was observed in the two comparison communities of Westerly and Newport. The rate of alcohol-related crashes with severe or fatal injury decreased in Woonsocket while the rate generally increased in the comparison communities (Figure 9.4), with predictable effects on hospital emergency room admissions.

Long-term follow-up evaluation demonstrated that these changes must be periodically reinforced. In particular, changing law enforcement priorities and police leadership resulted in loss of funding to apply the improved alcohol policy policing techniques (Stout *et al.*, 1992).

Contact

A detailed discussion of CAAIPP, including evaluation of its results, is found in Rhode Island Department of Health (1989) and in Harrington, Putnam, Waters, and Colt (1989). Additional information is available from William J. Waters, Jr., Ph.D., Rhode Island Department of Health, Cannon Building, 3 Capitol Hill, Providence, RI 02908-5097.

IGNITION INTERLOCK DEVICE TRIAL, OHIO

Police annually make over 1 million arrests for the crime of driving under the influence (DUI) of alcohol. Tougher laws requiring severe penalties do not appear to have a significant long-term effect on the problem. One prevention alternative is the use of an ignition interlock device to deter car owners convicted of DUI offenses from recurrent impaired driving. An interlock device connects an automobile ignition to a breath analyzer, effectively requiring drivers to take a blood alcohol concentration test every time they start the car.

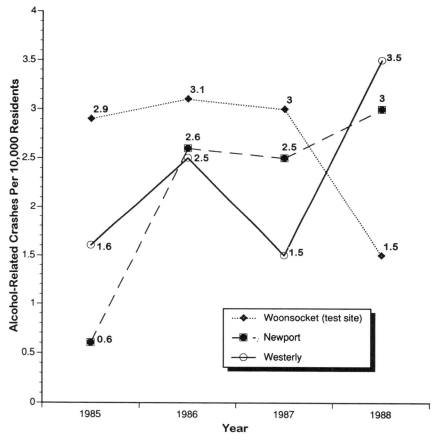

Figure 9.4. CAAIPP: rate of alcohol-related motor vehicle crashes with severe/fatal injury in three Rhode Island communities.

Origin

California's Farr-Davis Safety Act of 1986 was the first legislation to authorize use of the ignition interlock as a judicial response to DUI. By 1990, 16 states passed similar legislation.

Implementation

Ignition interlocks typically are offered as an alternative to license suspension after multiple convictions of DUI offenses or after a conviction of DUI that appears to be part of a history of other alcohol-related offenses. Installation of the device usually is accompanied by a sentence of a fine or jail term.

After installation, the driver must blow into a breath analyzer before turning the ignition key. If the analyzer indicates a blood alcohol concentration that exceeds a calibrated setting on the device, the car will not start. Drivers can circumvent the device by having a passenger blow into the analyzer. For example, some offenders have encouraged underaged children to accompany them in the car so that they can use the child's breath results to continue to drink and drive. The analyzer also can be disabled or avoided by driving another car that is not equipped with the device.

Outcome

The NIAAA sponsored an evaluation of the effectiveness of the devices in reducing recidivism of alcohol-impaired driving. Drivers convicted of DUI offenses in Hamilton County, Ohio (i.e., the city of Cincinnati and its suburbs), between July of 1987 and February of 1989 received a choice of license suspension or continued driving privileges with an ignition interlock device.[2]

Thirty months after the initial conviction, drivers with suspended licenses were three times more likely than drivers with an interlock device to have a subsequent DUI arrest (see Figure 9.5). In addition, they were ten times more likely to violate the court-ordered restriction (i.e., to drive without a license compared to circumventing the interlock device). The ignition interlock proved much more effective in preventing repeat DUI problems.

Contact

Details on the evaluation of interlock devices in Hamilton County are found in Morse and Elliott (1992). Barbara Morse, codirector of the study, is currently at the Institute of Behavioral Science, Box 442, University of Colorado, Boulder, CO 80309.

SELF-REGULATION TRAINING, VERMONT

Self-Regulation Training recruits beverage outlets to conduct community education targeting DUI. The education effort distributes drink calculators to help beverage purchasers make better decisions about the amount of alcohol con-

---

[2] According to reviews by Morse and Elliott (1992), low-income drivers and members of some ethnic groups appear more likely than other drivers to choose license suspension over the imposition of the interlock device.

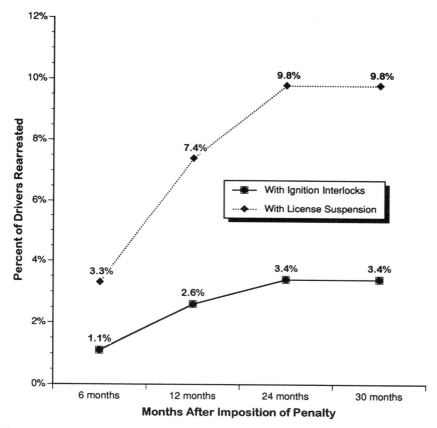

Figure 9.5. Ignition interlock device trial: comparison of DUI-convicted driver rearrest rates in Hamilton County, Ohio.

sumed. Drink calculators are inexpensive cardboard devices that estimate the blood alcohol concentration resulting from the number of drinks consumed for various body weights.

Origin

Drink calculators traditionally have been used in driver education courses. In 1983, the Office of Health Promotion Research of the University of Vermont, the state Alcoholic Beverage Commission, and the state Alcohol and Drug Abuse

Division collaborated on an assessment of the use of drink calculators in a community education program to reduce the prevalence of DUI offenses among the adult population.

Implementation

The experiment was held in a town of 3000 people with 25 retail alcoholic beverage outlets: convenience stores, restaurants, private clubs, filling stations, bars, supermarkets, and a state liquor store. Two types of drink calculators were offered at the outlets. Customer service personnel were trained in the use and benefits of the devices, and in appropriate education techniques for their clientele. No retail licensees refused to participate and roughly 6000 drink calculators were distributed.

Use of the devices also was demonstrated in public service spots airing approximately 20 times per week on a local television station. The public service announcements featured the community's bartenders and the area's most celebrated professional sports figure.

Outcome

Retail outlets in the community reported favorable responses and generally good acceptance of the drink calculators during a 6-month study period. Adult customers who purchased alcoholic beverages frequently were most likely to be exposed to the educational program and to receive one or more drink calculators.

After 6 months, the results of random screening of blood alcohol concentration of drivers in the community were compared with the results of similar screenings in a community that was exposed to the television spots without the retail outlet participation, and in a community where no intervention took place (Figure 9.6). The television spots had an apparent effect of reducing the percentage of drinkers who tested at blood alcohol concentration higher than 0.05, at which impairment begins. However, the combination of the retail outlet program with the television spots had a dramatic effect on the percentage of drivers who tested higher than 0.10, the state level for a DUI arrest at that time. Beverage distributors also developed positive feelings for the intervention because it made them partially responsible for preventing the more serious problems resulting from the use of their product.

The drink calculator program assumed that most people want to remain under the legal limit for DUI but lacked a means of objectively determining how much alcohol they can consume. The program may be less effective among underage drinkers, who lack access to the drink calculators because they cannot legally purchase beverages. It may also be less effective in states where laws against DUI prohibit any measurable alcohol use prior to driving.

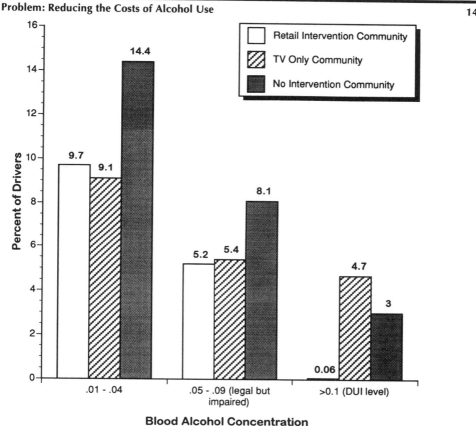

Figure 9.6. Self-Regulation Training: driver blood alcohol concentrations in follow-up survey.

Contact

A published account of the drink calculator experiment is found in Worden, Flynn, Merrill, Waller, and Haugh (1989). Dr. John K. Worden can be contacted at the Office of Health Promotion Research, University of Vermont, 1 South Prospect Street, Burlington, VT 05405.

TEAMS–GAMES–TOURNAMENTS, GEORGIA

Teams–Games–Tournaments (TGT) was a classroom-based education program emphasizing group tasks, designed specifically to influence the drinking and driving behavior of young adults after graduation from high school.

Origin

TGT was developed during the late 1970s and early 1980s by faculty of the University of Georgia, following extensive research in the use of games as teaching devices. Early applications of the health education technique included nutritional education (Wodarski, Adelson, Todd, & Wodarski, 1980). NHTSA and the University of Georgia Research Foundation contributed to field testing of the technique applied to prevention of alcohol-impaired driving.

Implementation

TGT required 50 minutes of daily class time for 4 weeks. Students are organized into eight-person teams; each team was designed to include members who received high, low, and average scores on a pretest on alcohol topics. The students were not informed of the pretest results. Teams studied as a group and competed in weekly tournaments on alcohol-related topics.

The curriculum emphasized self-management skills in addition to factors involved in irresponsible use of alcohol. These skills included assertiveness, refusal skills, and general problem solving techniques. Sessions were led by classroom teachers who completed a half-day training workshop.

Outcome

A long-term evaluation of program effects was conducted at several Georgia schools, comparing TGT participants to students in a traditional lecture-based alcohol education program and to students who received no educational program. The comparisons included self-reported alcohol-related behavior as well as knowledge and attitudes pertaining to alcohol use (Wodarski, 1987).

Program participants dramatically improved in knowledge and prosocial attitudes concerning alcohol use. They also exhibited general improvement in self-reported drinking behavior. Statistically significant differences between program graduates and the two comparison groups continued to be observed 2 years later (see Figure 9.7). The curriculum thus demonstrated success in influencing alcohol behavior after graduation. More significantly, the 2-year follow-up also demonstrated that traditional alcohol education represented only a marginal improvement over failing to provide any alcohol education at all.

Contact

The most detailed published description of TGT is found in Wodarski (1987). No current contact has been identified and the curriculum does not appear to be available.

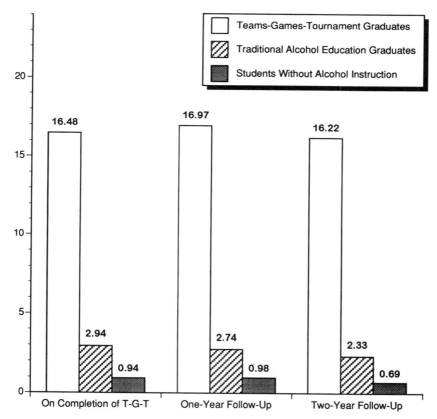

Figure 9.7. Teams–Games–Tournaments: drinking and driving test scores of TGT graduates and two high school senior control groups.

UNIVERSITY STUDENT ALCOHOL INTERVENTION, ════ WASHINGTON

College fraternities, sororities, and dormitories are infamous as breeding grounds for alcohol-related problems. As described earlier, campus life is often a first experience in unsupervised living and freshmen may be unprepared for the intense pressure to drink too much too often. As early as the Renaissance, for example, Germany's Heidelberg University maintained a private jail for drunken students.

Colleges have long sought to identify effective interventions for students who exhibit alcohol-related problems. Such students are usually not long-established alcoholics. In fact, anecdotal evidence suggests that young people with no high school alcohol experience are most vulnerable to developing serious alcohol problems in the college environment. Recent efforts have found that a diagnosis of alcoholism is seldom appropriate while mass education of the incoming freshman class is too diffuse to address serious cases. The University of Washington performed experimental trials to assess other methods for reducing alcohol abuse among college-aged youth and young adults.

Origin

Professor G. Alan Marlatt of the University of Washington has maintained a consistent interest in the effectiveness of interventions for individuals who do not have the symptoms of alcohol dependence but are encountering significant problems resulting from "learned" inappropriate alcohol consumption. The University of Washington student alcohol interventions were established as a series of clinical trials supported by the NIAAA.

Implementation

Three types of intervention were made available to students who had experienced at least one alcohol-related problem, as defined by a standardized diagnostic instrument; the average age of participants in the controlled experiment was 21. Two intervention formats emphasized the development of self-monitoring skills, either through six weekly group sessions or through use of a self-help manual. The third intervention format consisted of a single session of professional advice and interpersonal counseling. Similar "brief interventions" have become a popular alternative to long-term alcoholism counseling among clients who do not appear alcohol-dependent.

Outcome

Two years after the intervention, most participants in both the professional advice and group session formats had significantly reduced their alcohol consumption, as measured by peak estimated blood alcohol level, weekly drinking patterns, and monthly total consumption (see Figure 9.8). No similar results were obtained for the individual approach using the self-help manual.

The experiments suggest that brief interventions among young adults experiencing alcohol-related problems can prevent more serious problems and reduce future needs for treatment and/or justice system intervention. They also suggest that merely providing information on self-monitoring skills, without

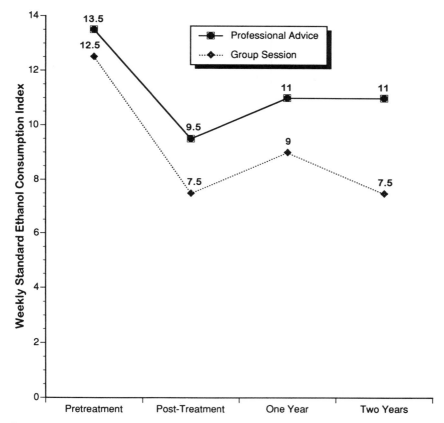

Figure 9.8. University of Washington intervention participants: change in average weekly ethanol (alcohol) consumption.

additional intervention, is not enough to affect the long-term behavior of most college-educated drinkers.

Contacts

A good description of the experiment is included in Baer, Kivlahan, Fromme, and Marlatt (1991). More recent information is available from Professor G. Alan Marlatt and Dr. Mary Larimer, Addictive Behaviors Research Center, Department of Psychology, Box 351525, University of Washington, Seattle, WA 98195.

GENERAL OBSERVATIONS

Americans have made a conscious decision to legalize only one intoxicating drug. When they repealed the Noble Experiment of prohibition of alcoholic beverages, the people of the United States indicated that they were prepared to pay a price in exchange for the freedom to drink alcohol. The costs to society of alcohol abuse, however, rose more rapidly than anyone anticipated. In particular, the healthcare costs related to frequent drinking, to alcohol-impaired driving and boating, and to the violence and sexual license that often accompanies intoxication now represent perhaps as much as 20% of the total medical expenses of the United States.

Fortunately, alcohol-related problems appear to be very susceptible to prevention measures. Societal norms regarding alcohol use have been moving in the direction of lower consumption and intolerance of obvious drunkenness. The three-martini business lunch of the 1960s is now seen as a dysfunctional behavior rather than a necessity for successful marketing; even the classic cocktail party may not survive the 20th century.

Responsible beverage service training, school-based curricula, effective enforcement of laws restricting alcohol misuse, and the brief interventions that proved successful with problem drinkers at the University of Seattle accept a legitimate role for alcoholic beverages in society. All of these interventions can contribute to further reducing the healthcare costs and human tragedies associated with permitting Americans to drink alcoholic beverages. In addition, they all are based on the assumption that adults will rationally choose to limit their alcohol use when provided with accurate information, timely cues, and credible legal threats.

However, none of these interventions are free. When communities fail to budget for enforcement of laws and regulations related to alcohol use, when schools decide that driver education focusing on the dangers of alcohol-impaired driving is an expendable luxury, and when server intervention training is seen as a one-time effort, the costs of alcohol use invariably rise. The choice always is to pay a small amount for effective prevention now or pay much more for our society's legal intoxicant later.

Problem: Organizing the Community for Prevention

After 70 years, the public now recognizes infectious disease control as "belonging" to the local health department, water quality to the public works department, and blood supply to the Red Cross. Substance abuse prevention, in contrast, lacks a traditional organizational home in the community infrastructure. Instead, every community has been expected to create its own structure for drug abuse prevention with little or no guidance from historical experience, but with lots of advice on the need to be "participatory" or "stakeholder-driven." Without an overall structure, however, substance abuse prevention is guaranteed to be wasteful and inefficient simply because so many groups are willing to independently finance and organize potentially competing prevention efforts.

Organizing the community for prevention can be bloody. Agencies and interest groups that claim the title of the "natural" managers of prevention include health departments, neighborhood associations, law enforcement agencies, charities, ethnic affinity groups, child welfare agencies, the parent movement, schools, and private business. Like participants in a nasty child custody fight who focus on winning rather than the child's interests, well-intentioned groups sometimes seem to lose sight of the needs of effective prevention in the midst of squabbling over formal responsibilities.

The findings of demonstration projects organized by the federal Center for Substance Abuse Prevention (CSAP) suggest that *who* runs prevention may be less important for effective results than ensuring that each participating agency has a suitable, well-defined role. A national cross-site evaluation of 251 substance abuse prevention partnerships sponsored by CSAP found that turf conflicts were cited as a barrier to the achievement of community anti-drug abuse goals in 45% of the partnerships (Center for Substance Abuse Prevention, 1995).

SELECTING A MODEL FOR PREVENTION INFRASTRUCTURE

Selecting an appropriate model for prevention infrastructure is similar to deciding what model car to purchase. Affordability is an issue: A large, complex permanent organization costs more money than a simpler structure. Regular maintenance can also be an issue because complicated decision-making processes require frequent face-to-face meetings among the decision makers. Of course, even the simplest structures for making community decisions on drug abuse prevention demand periodic inspection and an occasional organizational tune-up. Above all, the infrastructure selected for a prevention effort must be roomy enough to accommodate everyone who will be providing a leadership role. A small town that opts to focus prevention activities on adolescents may be able to operate its program effectively with the organizational equivalent of a subcompact car: a standing committee with representatives from the school system, the police, and the healthcare system, with such nonprofit groups as the churches, the PTA, and the local youth organizations providing permanent observers. A statewide or regional prevention coalition, in contrast, may need to have comfortable organizational "leg room" for dozens of participants.

The four programs highlighted in this chapter specifically examined how to organize the structural environment for effective prevention of alcohol and drug abuse among adolescents. Two programs operated at the neighborhood level, one implemented prevention throughout a metropolitan area, and the fourth organized a small town. The organizational sophistication varied, depending on the scope of the effort and the size of the community served. In each case, however, the leadership understood that substance abuse prevention demands a coherent structure that allows decisions to be based on a thorough understanding of the target population.

SPECIALIZATION BY CLIENT TYPE: THE CADRE PROJECT, CALIFORNIA

The CADRE project originated with the Department of Health of the City of San Francisco, the traditional local source of expertise for public health promotion and disease prevention. Most clients were youth aged 12 to 18 who lived in San Francisco neighborhoods characterized by high rates of drug use, alcohol abuse, and drug-related HIV infection.

Origin

CADRE was created in 1987 as a demonstration project for funding by CSAP. It combined and expanded existing youth outreach programs in substance abuse, HIV, and pregnancy prevention.

CADRE's principal activities were chosen by the Department of Public Health. Other groups were made contractually responsible for implementing prevention activities for a specific subgroups of clients:

- Elementary school youth and parents—the local affiliate of the National Council on Alcoholism
- Youth involved in drug use but not in the juvenile justice system—13 neighborhood agencies, including a public high school and a local hospital
- Youth involved in the juvenile justice system—a single designated community mental health center

This method of organizing prevention services required each provider to develop expertise in outreach and operations with its "own" constituency.

Differences in services provided to the three populations reflected community advocacy for critical unmet needs among each of the groups. Among younger children, the project provided classroom education on social skills, assertiveness, and learning skills. The health department recognized that it erred by not having family intervention from the outset and eventually provided family support groups.

Older youth received peer counseling and classroom education on drug abuse and HIV. Youth who were adjudicated under the juvenile justice system received more intensive counseling, drug education, and case management. Other components of the project included strengthened interagency prevention linkages.

CADRE's experience was helpful in the planning for neighborhood revitalization programs in two business districts of San Francisco. The focus in these revitalization efforts was to recruit the business communities to participate in community wellness and anticrime efforts that would make the targeted neighborhoods safer for people to shop in. Small businesses organized to sponsor health fairs, street art fairs for local youth, and improved street lighting. The most dramatic episode was the organization of a sit-in by local merchants at a lunch counter known to be a gathering place for drug dealers. Over time, the business initiative suffered from leadership burnout, but participants claimed to be pleased with the results.

Over a period of 1 year, data collection from youth street samples in the targeted communities found statistically significant changes in knowledge and attitudes related to AIDS and substance abuse, and a statistically significant reduction in the use of specific drugs among 12- to 18-year-olds, with the sharpest declines among African-American youth. The neighborhood revitalization activities with the business community produced a reduction in the visibility of drug problems in the area, increased retail sales volume, and reduced crime.

Contact

Information on these programs was derived from unpublished reports submitted by the Department of Public Health of San Francisco to the Center for Substance Abuse Prevention in 1988–90. For additional information on CADRE, contact Wayne Clark, Ph.D., San Francisco Department of Public Health, 1380 Howard Street, San Francisco, CA 94103. For information on the neighborhood revitalization effort, contact the Mayor's Community Partnership Program, City Hall, Room 2A, San Francisco, CA 94102.

SPECIALIZATION BY FUNCTION: GREATER ALLIANCE FOR PREVENTION SYSTEM, ILLINOIS

GAPS was a neighborhood consortium that emphasized changing the community norms to be more intolerant of substance abuse. GAPS also worked directly with African-American youth, developing social competency and providing activities to instill cultural pride. The consortium divided responsibilities for youth activities among agencies by function rather than by client type.

Origin

The consortium model of organizing services was one of the first to be evaluated by a federal drug abuse prevention agency. The staff of the Bobby E. Wright Mental Health Center in Chicago, in collaboration with the Illinois Department of Alcohol and Substance Abuse, organized GAPS in response to the announcement of a federal service demonstration grant in 1987.

Implementation

The lead agency in GAPS recruited community groups to participate in community forums and vigils against substance abuse, and to educate adult residents about zoning violations committed by alcohol sales outlets. As in the San Francisco neighborhood revitalization initiative, staff of consortium member agencies were encouraged to directly confront local drug dealers.

In addition to efforts to the change the neighborhood environment, each agency in the consortium was assigned a specific task with teenagers and their parents:

- The African American Heritage Project recruited youth for drama performances and other activities to heighten interest in cultural heritage.
- Garfield Counseling Center provided life skills and peer leadership training.
- Prevention Partnership, Inc. assisted parent volunteers to develop and carry out anti-drug abuse action plans.
- Hispanic Alcoholism Services conducted workshops on alcohol and drug issues, and served as a local clearinghouse for drug information.

All GAPS services, however, were united under a single planning structure and a coalitionwide logo. Community members recognized that they were being served by GAPS rather than by the separate agencies.

Outcome

An outcome evaluation of GAPS was conducted in 1990 by faculty of the University of Illinois. After 1 year, 147 neighborhood teenagers who were highly involved in GAPS activities indicated statistically significant mean reduction in risk for tobacco and alcohol use, and a smaller reduction in risk of marijuana use. Teenagers who were less frequently involved in GAPS activities averaged no similar change in risk for alcohol or tobacco use, but tended to *increase* their risk for marijuana use (see Figure 10.1).

Statistically significant improvements among the high-involvement group also were indicated in assertiveness and cultural pride. These changes were associated with a hardening of participant attitudes against drug use. Similar changes in attitude were not observed among the comparison group of low-involvement youth residing in the service area. In effect, more intensive involvement by teenagers in the activities operated by the member agencies of the consortium was associated with significantly reduced risk for drug use, including both alcohol and marijuana use, and other positive changes.

Contact

Information on the GAPS consortium was derived from unpublished reports submitted by the Bobby Wright Neighborhood Center to CSAP in 1988–90, and from an unpublished program evaluation prepared by faculty of the University of Illinois at Urbana–Champaign, in July, 1990. Evaluation data on the GAPS

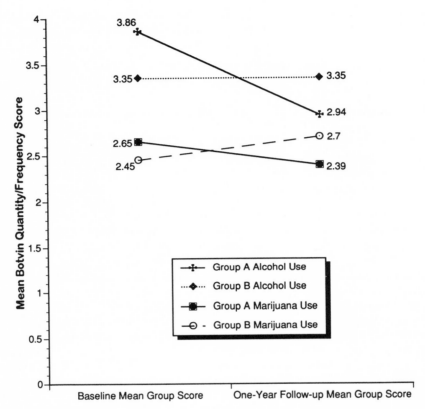

Figure 10.1. GAPS Project: Mean frequency/quantity use scores for selected substances among teenagers in project service area (higher scores indicate increased use). Group A—teenage residents participating in GAPS activities. Group B—teenage residents with little or no involvement in GAPS activities.

consortium are available from Dr. Jean E. Rhodes, Department of Psychology, University of Illinois at Urbana–Champaign, 603 East Daniel Street, Champaign, IL 61820.

TOP-DOWN PLANNING: MIDWEST PREVENTION PROGRAM/ PROJECT STAR

The Midwest Prevention Program (MPP) is one of the best-known experiments in drug abuse prevention. MPP was designed as a methodologically rigorous test to determine the effects of a complex, metropolitan area-wide drug abuse prevention structure. In addition, the designers of the program wanted to see if their creation could be duplicated in more than one city. For this reason, MPP phased-in similar school and community activities over several years in Kansas City, Missouri, and Indianapolis, Indiana.

Origin

The research design and schedule of activities of MPP were developed principally by Drs. C. Anderson Johnson and Mary Ann Pentz of the University of Southern California School of Medicine in 1983–84. The social influences model, in which prevention is fostered by combining social skills with the development of an environment that is hostile to drug use, supplied the theoretical basis for the MPP. A phased introduction of activities was key to the study design.

Support for the project was provided initially by the National Institute on Drug Abuse, the Ewing Marion Kauffman Foundation, the Lilly Endowment, and the pharmaceutical manufacturing firm of Marion Merrell Dow, Inc. The Kansas City component of MPP was also known as Project STAR (Students Taught Awareness and Resistance), and received additional funding from the U.S. Department of Education, local school systems, and private sponsors. The Indianapolis component was known as Project I-STAR. I-STAR received support from private contributors and from the U.S. Department of Housing and Urban Development.

Implementation

The MPP featured three important differences from most community-based prevention efforts:

- MPP was implemented according to a set schedule of phased-in activities, starting with media events during the first year and continuing through the regulatory policy changes planned by the prevention task force in the sixth and final year.
- Key planning decisions for STAR and I-STAR were made by the University of Southern California research team, with local groups concentrating their efforts on the details of implementation.
- MPP crossed jurisdictional lines to include every school district in the metropolitan area.

A well-planned publicity campaign, focusing on recruiting the support of the news media, preceded the implementation of specific prevention activities.

Extensive news coverage of the project was viewed as essential to a favorable climate for prevention efforts and to recruitment of parents, volunteers, and local officials.

The educational element of MPP began with a ten-session classroom program for grades 6 and 7, designed by the Institute for Prevention Research at the University of Southern California. Ninth-grade students received a booster session.

Classroom assignments included "homework" to foster parent involvement. Additional adult activities included a Parent Skills Program, based on training parent volunteers to deliver a curriculum in their home community on the following:

- Identifying school and community needs
- Reinforcing resistance skills
- Positive friendships
- Enhancing communications skills (e.g., attentive listening and communicating expectations)
- Setting and enforcing rules

MPP also organized adult volunteers into eight Action Committees, each representing different segments of the community (e.g., Media, Medical/Treatment, Parent/Family, Religious). Action Committees served as advisors to the project staff on implementation and formed a preventive health task force to develop policies affecting the community environment.

Outcome

Evaluations of the MPP began with students in eight Kansas City public schools, then expanded to include all of the Kansas City and Indianapolis metropolitan areas. Three years after the first classroom sessions, students from program and control schools exhibited significant differences in the likelihood of tobacco or marijuana use during the past 30 days (Figure 10.2). By 1990, self-reports and carbon dioxide testing found mean tobacco, marijuana, and alcohol use was 20 to 40% lower among 12th graders exposed to the program than among nonparticipants (e.g., see Pentz *et al.* 1991).

Contacts

Published sources on the MPP include Pentz *et al.* (1989a,b), and MacKinnon *et al.* (1991). The project director, Professor Mary A. Pentz, can be contacted at

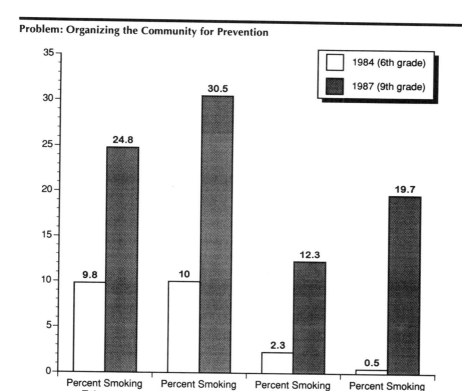

Figure 10.2. MPP: 30-day prevalence of smoking among initial cohort 3 years after intervention.

the Institute for Prevention Research, University of Southern California, 1540 Alcazar Street, CHP 207, Pasadena, CA 90033.

LOW-TECH LINKAGES: UPPER LITTLE CAILLOU DRUG-FREE SCHOOL, LOUISIANA

Chauvin, Louisiana is a small town near the Gulf of Mexico, 80 miles southwest of New Orleans. Alcohol abuse is by far the most widespread adolescent substance abuse problem in the area, perhaps reflecting traditional tolerance for alcohol-laden celebration among the largely French-speaking population.

Upper Little Caillou School in Chauvin overcame obstacles of isolation, the absence of direct federal or foundation grants, and initial lack of local concern about teenage alcohol use, to build a successful prevention program. The solution to most of these challenges was the development of effective prevention linkages between the school and the surrounding community.

Origin

The Upper Little Caillou program was developed through the Drug-Free School and Communities Program (later Safe and Drug-Free Schools Program) of the U.S. Department of Education. The program provided grants to the states, which then passed the funds through to local school districts such as Terrebonne Parish.

When declining oil revenue during the late 1980s appeared to increase crime and alcohol abuse rates in southern Louisiana, the school embarked on a program to increase its influence through an expanded community presence for the Drug-Free School and Communities Program. The University of Oklahoma, as Drug-Free School Resource Center for the southwestern United States until 1996, provided technical assistance and training.

Implementation

School staff began community outreach with a campaign to increase awareness of the costs to Chauvin from underage alcohol use. The staff emphasized education on the effects of teenage drinking on academic performance (and possibilities for future employment), impaired driving, and the potential for an increase in other drug use.

The school used its share of the Drug-Free and Communities grant to acquire curricula and information materials. At the same time, school staff held informal meetings with parents, law enforcement officials, and business owners to discuss how existing local resources could be used to support prevention activities. The results included tighter enforcement of laws against alcohol sales to minors, business in-kind contributions to alcohol-free social events, and parent fund-raising to finance a school trip to New Orleans. Many of the more innovative fund-raising events received extensive publicity, including coverage by a New Orleans-based TV news broadcast.

The New Orleans trip was the first time many of the students in Chauvin had ever left the county. Principal Betty Peltier believes that it was crucial for the program success to expose youth to the possibilities beyond their rural community.

━━━ **Outcome**

Five years after beginning the community outreach, self-reports among high school seniors indicated a 15 to 30% decrease in mean quantity and frequency of alcohol use, and smaller decreases in marijuana use.

━━━ **Contact**

Information on the Upper Little Caillou program is derived from unpublished reports presented to the Annual Symposium, Southwest Region Drug-Free Schools and Communities, Albuquerque, May, 1993. Additional information is available from the staff of Upper Little Caillou School under the direction of Betty Peltier, Principal, Chauvin, LA 70344.

━━━━━━━━━━━━━━━━━━━━━━━━━━━━━━━━━━━━━━ **GENERAL OBSERVATIONS**

In each case described in this chapter, the organizers of the prevention services chose a structure that included key groups in the planning process. Crucial decisions on the content of the prevention program, however, were retained under central control by people with specific training on substance abuse issues. This mix of expert guidance on *what* to do, when coupled with community participation in discussions on *how* to do it, seems to be a winning combination regardless of the type of agency responsible for managing the operation.

Another important component of a successful prevention coalition appears to be having a written plan or set of guidelines on what activities and goals are to be accomplished by the organization. This is more likely to occur when government officials are not in the driver's seat, according to a nationwide survey by the Join Together project of the Robert Wood Johnson Foundation (Join Together, 1996). Government agencies, including school systems, are locked into budget and activity priorities by legislative mandates and complex appropriation process; they generally lack the flexibility to engage in long-term strategic planning. For this reason, most prevention advocates recommend a public–private partnership as the most effective approach to organizing community prevention services.

A final component that appears to help the success of organizing for substance abuse prevention is the development of solid relationships with the news media. The MPP, the Upper Little Caillou drug-free schools effort, and CADRE all benefited from favorable publicity generated by program organizers actively seeking coverage by newspapers and broadcasters. The Upper Little Caillou program in particular displayed a high level of creativity and perseverance in drawing attention to its activities, from offering samples of the local delicacy of seafood gumbo to the audience at national presentations, to preparing a gigantic sheet cake that both raised money and provided an unusual pictorial story for the TV cameras. News coverage translates into community awareness and support for the prevention organization, and that increased level of support permits more activities that should generate more news coverage.

Tiresome details on decision-making processes, preparation of a written strategy statement, and the care and feeding of the news media may seem to be distant from the core objective of trying to stop substance abuse. Such details, however, ultimately make the difference between a prevention effort that can be sustained over time and a program that dies as soon as its sponsor or founder moves on to other concerns.

A Short "To Do" List for Drug Abuse Prevention

The variety of solutions to reduce substance abuse problems presented in the preceding chapters may be somewhat disconcerting to a reader who expected this book to include a single blueprint for successful prevention. No single set of activities is automatically the "right" approach to prevention of the most frequently encountered problems of alcohol abuse and drug use. Instead, communities have lots of choices to make among activities that protect their residents from substance abuse.

The fact that several combinations of activities contribute to prevention is a boon for communities concerned about drug abuse. Consider the alternative, namely, that consistently successful drug use prevention among adolescents might demand, for example, a week-long wilderness challenge combined with intensive interpersonal counseling. Under such conditions, the only jurisdictions able to offer effective prevention to teenagers would be those that could afford field trips and professional counselors. Instead, successful drug abuse prevention can rely on combinations of activities available to most communities. Programs producing significant results among inner-city youth do not require busing to the nearest wilderness or a platoon of licensed clinical social workers. Similarly, prevention for young children in a sparsely populated rural county does not demand a well-run neighborhood drop-in center. Effective drug abuse prevention depends on making good choices for the local environment rather than duplicating someone else's successful program.

Given the importance of choosing among activities that produce results, the key problem for communities trying to reduce drug abuse is learning how to be a careful consumer of prevention services. This may be the one area in prevention in which most policymakers fail. Bluntly stated, otherwise intelligent people often exercise poor judgment in choosing a mix of activities that is supposed to reduce drug abuse in their community.

Table 11.1 illustrates that decision strategies that are clearly inappropriate for careful purchase of a new car seem to acquire legitimacy when applied to

Table 11.1. Examples of Ineffective Decision-Making Applied to New Car Purchase and to Selection of Drug Abuse Prevention

Decision-making strategy	As applied to a new car purchase	Applied to selecting activities for drug use prevention
Rely on advice from respected but unqualified "expert"	Purchase based on comments of co-worker or cousin who owns similar model	Selection deferred to parent group members or community activists with no training or experience in prevention
Rely on celebrity endorsement	Purchase based on ads featuring Indy 500 winner or sports figure driving the car	Selection determined by endorsement of professional group or by locally influential figure, e.g., police chief
Cost factor dominance	Purchase based on low price or easy credit ("low money down; no payment due 'til next year")	Selection based on availability of grant funds or on low start-up cost
Glamor and head-turning appeal	Purchase based on styling details or on glossy brochure or advertisements	Selection based on attractive packaging of curriculum or slick marketing
Random chance selection	Purchase of first car seen on the lot or selection based on a coin flip	Selection made with no systematic review of alternatives

selecting a drug abuse prevention program. For example, drug education curricula often are marketed using the techniques used to sell commercial products. Officials who resist high-pressure sales gimmicks offered by other types of vendors often turn gullible when similar tactics are used to convince them to acquire a drug abuse prevention program.

A grant to conduct a specific type of prevention activity illustrates how decisions on drug abuse prevention may become distorted. The source of the grant may be well intentioned but armed with an agenda that does not conform to the community's needs. The risk of an inappropriate agenda is obvious when a brewery funds community prevention of alcohol-related problems; however, it is equally possible when a scientist proposes to test a theory of prevention by running a time-limited controlled experiment in a local public school.

The suggestions in this chapter apply to the problem of choosing among prevention options. Support for these suggestions is based largely on experiences of the Fighting Back grants of the Robert Wood Johnson Foundation and the recipients of grants from CSAP's Community Prevention Partnership program. Adherence to these suggestions does not guarantee successful prevention results, but can help communities make better choices.

BASE PREVENTION PRIORITIES ON NEED

Use of specific drugs is not uniform across all communities. Comparing drug-related emergencies in three metropolitan areas (see Figure 11.1) reveals that some areas, such as Boston and Seattle, have been centers for the abuse of heroin, while other cities, including Atlanta, have no significant heroin problems. This doesn't necessarily mean that cities with few heroin users were havens from drug abuse: Atlanta area drug users, in contrast, appear to have favored cocaine.

Such differences in drug use among communities are not accidents. Patterns of drug trafficking and availability, law enforcement, demography, economic prosperity, and cultural traditions also influence drug use within a given community. Heroin, for example, is more widespread in New Mexico than in North Dakota because the drug is more likely to be smuggled from Mexico than from Canada. Inhaling chemicals to become intoxicated is a major problem in the farm belt where the chemicals are easily accessible but is much less of a problem in the inner city.

Drug abuse prevention is never cost-effective when targeted at a behavior that doesn't represent a major problem. For example, one large suburban school district invested much of its antidrug budget in "sniffer" dogs to detect drugs in high school lockers. Surprise afterschool sweeps of every building produced no drug samples. During the same period, students from the school district were

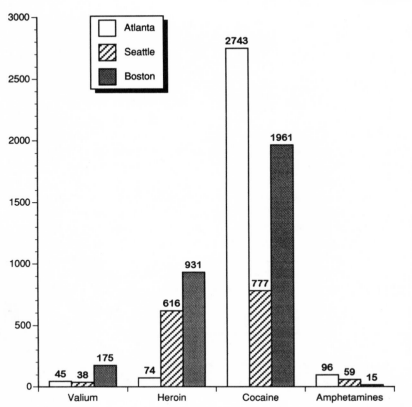

Figure 11.1. Emergency room admissions for selected drugs in three metropolitan areas, 1990. Source: National Institute on Drug Abuse. (1991). *Annual emergency room data 1990—Data from the Drug Abuse Warning Network* (Series 1, No. 10-A). Rockville, MD: National Institute on Drug Abuse.

arrested for distributing LSD at parties. A survey to identify *where* drugs were abused by the suburban teenagers could have saved thousands of dollars wasted in the locker search—and perhaps would have been better invested in school-based prevention efforts on LSD.

The Strengthening Black Families Program in Selma, Alabama, described in Chapter 3 is an example of appropriate targeting. Selma chose to address a drug problem that involved relatively few people but major potential future costs. The resulting prevention program, despite a high per person price tag, may have been the most cost-effective prevention investment possible for the small town.

Recent progress in the prevention field has simplified the process of conducting a needs assessment for local drug control. The Regional Drug

Initiative in Portland, Oregon, pioneered development of a Drug Impact Index to document the scope of drug problems in a community. The Robert Wood Johnson's Join Together program also produced a handbook that helps to quantify specific problems. These techniques, based on such data as arrest records and hospital admissions, can be supplemented with survey research to produce a detailed picture of community prevention needs.

Implementation of a needs assessment in a small community requires some expertise for the sake of credibility, but does not depend on hiring costly outside consultants. The entire needs assessment package can be performed as a group assignment by a class in social science methodology at a local university under the direction of a competent faculty member, or by volunteers from the research department of a locally based corporation. A needs assessment team can obtain guidance either from the Regional Drug Initiative at 522 SW 5th Street, Suite 1310, Portland, OR 97204, or from Join Together at 441 Stuart Street, Boston, MA 02116.

MATCH INTERVENTIONS WITH POPULATIONS

Scattered throughout the previous discussions of specific prevention efforts are examples of programs that had impressive outcomes for some populations and virtually no effects on other populations. Thus, Self-Regulation Training in Vermont as described in Chapter 9 was no more effective than television spots at reducing the percentage of light-drinking drivers, but was very effective at deterring drivers from drinking in excess of the DUI limit. Similarly, the outcomes for the AMPS curriculum described in Chapter 5 documented effects on teenage drinking only (1) when introduced in sixth grade rather than fifth grade and (2) when participants already had experimented with alcoholic beverages.

One reason why it is important to match populations with appropriate interventions is that people do not learn the same way when they are young children as when they are teenagers or adults. They also are not motivated by identical concerns. The child of an alcoholic or the survivor of a dysfunctional home environment does not perceive the same world as the product of a stable, sober household. Previous experience with alcohol or drugs seems to be another factor that shapes perception of prevention messages. These differences in learning style and world view have a strong impact on how to best prevent drug use behavior among different groups.

People differ in other ways that affect prevention results. Cultural variables also appear to affect implementation of a well-designed prevention program. The prevention community has invested significant effort in researching "cultural competence" in prevention messages; the importance of this sometimes may be overstated, but there is no question that a good program that ignores the culture of the population served risks becoming ineffective. In one classic case, a school system with a large minority population selected a prevention curriculum that focused on Afrocentric values—forgetting that the content might not appeal to members of a growing contingent of students of Puerto Rican ancestry. An evaluation by an African-American evaluator found that most of the students of Puerto Rican ancestry were in fact hostile to the prevention program because it was described as "promoting African values."

There is no reason why communities and health service providers must choose one program of prevention for everyone. The best prevention policy is one that recognizes the differences between groups and selects appropriate interventions for each population. Selection of priority target populations for drug abuse prevention should be a first step toward deciding what programs will be applied to which groups.

INVENTORY WHAT'S IN PLACE

After selecting the interventions, organizers of a drug abuse prevention effort should soberly list every resource that the interventions will need to be effective and then identify where in the community the resource can be found. This inventory process may cause the planners to revisit their choices, or it may suggest new possibilities. At the very least, it will indicate which resources must be purchased and which can be acquired by other means.

In 1987, a community foundation in Washington, D.C. decided to earmark $50,000 in drug abuse prevention interventions for youth at the highest risk for serious drug involvement. Its leadership developed a model that required case management for the youth, substance abuse education for both African-American and Central American immigrant adolescents, drug-free recreational activities, and intensive counseling to resolve family problems and help clients navigate the child welfare system. The foundation could have spent considerable time and money hiring the personnel and acquiring the other resources needed to carry out this ambitious program. Instead, it found that three nonprofit groups individually were providing Afrocentric and Hispanic drug education, and intensive counseling and advocacy for dysfunctional families. It also systematically contacted martial arts instructors and found several willing to donate 2 hours per week to teaching judo to boys or self-defense techniques to girls. The foundation recruited the three nonprofit groups as "subcontractors," paying a small stipend to compensate for the additional case load, and focused its own resources on developing the case management system and scheduling the martial arts instruction. The result was an initiative that provided a year of services to more than 1500 youth at a cost below $400 per participant.

The project described above did not produce outcomes that were sufficiently impressive to be included in this work, but it demonstrates the principle that drug abuse prevention does not need to own the resources it uses. Communities often are rich in programs, expertise, and materials that can be applied to prevention of drug problems. The National Guard, for example, may have the transport and the chaperones needed for a wilderness challenge outing. The Boy Scouts may be willing to lend a campsite and equipment for a therapeutic retreat. The Sunday school classroom at the church can be a perfect site for parent education and the cable TV company probably has facilities that can be lent for a one-time video training session.

INVEST MONEY AND EXPERTISE

Effective prevention of drug abuse is cheaper than treatment and is very much cheaper than the costs of an epidemic of drug use. However, as stated repeatedly, prevention is not free. It takes time and money to plan, schedule, and carry out a systematic program to prevent drug abuse. Sometimes policy changes, such as raising the minimum drinking age or banning the sale of drug use paraphernalia, are described as "cost-free." In fact, such policy changes actually carry invisible price tags in the form of court costs and other enforcement costs, and publicity about the change to inform the public that the policy is in effect.

Effective prevention also demands the services of capable and knowledgeable individuals to design and implement activities and interventions. Communities attempting to recruit and retain high-caliber talent for prevention efforts are competing against other potential employers. Substance abuse prevention programs on tribal land, for example, reputedly lose key college-educated personnel to the attractions of better-paying careers off the reservation. Although volunteers are a great asset that can stretch a small investment, they are no substitute for offering competitive salaries and job security to any permanent staff that the prevention effort needs.

The issue of prevention resources raises the question of ownership of prevention programs. A few of the prevention efforts described in this work have been copyrighted and require permission to use. In some cases, copyright may be filed to protect the integrity and reputation of the program; for example, to prevent a shady entrepreneur from misappropriating the name "D.A.R.E." for products that have nothing to do with the well-known prevention curriculum. In other cases, copyright permission may provide the only compensation for a prevention specialist's long hours of work in developing a program. The law requires respect for copyright protection. Charges for use rights are part of the legitimate expenses for prevention.

The existence of long-term charges for use rights and personnel demands a stable source of funds. Short-term funding opportunities are potentially useful for jump-starting prevention activities. Grant funds are used by successful programs to develop curricula, to design interventions and evaluations, and to conduct community outreach that wins support for prevention. Short-term grants also are helpful in training the people who eventually implement the program.

But grants do not provide long-term funding. The typical grant award from the federal government traditionally has been limited to 3 to 5 years. Foundation grants rarely have longer duration and United Way funding varies annually. These mechanisms cannot ensure a stable base for drug abuse prevention, any more than a community should expect short-term grants to fund restaurant inspection for prevention of food-borne disease.

The inability of grants to sustain prevention means that more stable sources of funding must be found. California, for example, has dedicated a portion of the state tax on cigarettes to be used for prevention of tobacco use. Many states have legislated that part of the proceeds from the sale of alcoholic beverages should be used for prevention of alcohol abuse. The local share of revenue from forfeiture of drug dealer properties also can be used for prevention, if the appropriate law enforcement agency agrees.

In Mobile, Alabama, the local prevention effort recruited the Mobile Gas Company as an organizer of voluntary contributions: Utility customers have the option of checking off on their gas bill a monthly donation to the community drug abuse prevention council. The result is a stable income of approximately $45,000 per year that does not require grant applications, annual appropriations, or a major voluntary fund-raising effort.

In effect, when a community first attempts to define a comprehensive prevention effort, questions that must be asked include:

■ How will prevention be paid for in the long term?
■ How much money can be expected from these sources?
■ What effort can be sustained by these funds?

The Upper Little Caillou drug-free school program described in Chapter 10 provides a good example of a prevention effort that identified and secured resources from its community and built its effort around affordable activities. The program transformed the challenge of fund-raising for prevention from an unpleasant reality to one of the strengths of the intervention.

— **CALL THE DOCTOR**

A few people are obsessed about their physical well-being all of the time. Most of us, however, think about our bodies and wellness only when something is wrong. This is a problem for substance abuse prevention and promotion of behavioral health because the antidrug message frequently reaches the audience whose thoughts are focused elsewhere. Couch potatoes watching television generally are not thinking about health issues when an antidrug public service announcement flashes on the screen, commuters riding the bus are not focused on community substance abuse risks when they see a poster advertising the local drug abuse council, and even fifth-grade students attending a D.A.R.E. class may be looking ahead toward recess.

The ideal time to influence the health behavior of an individual is during the rare moment when she is concerned enough about health to do something about it. That moment usually comes when we visit the doctor, the dentist, the nurse, or the pharmacist. These professionals are credible sources of information pledged to promote patient health. Primary care clinicians and pediatricians, at least in theory, should be very influential in encouraging patients to avoid alcohol abuse and illegal drug use.

In the past, the experience of involving doctors in drug abuse prevention has fallen short of its potential. Most drug abuse prevention efforts do not try to systematically recruit medical professionals in the community other than a few individual doctors to serve as token representatives of their field. Clinicians rarely have the time to seek out the prevention field. Prevention activists often are surprised that clinicians have little formal training on the subject of illegal drugs, and medical professionals often are disgruntled by the lack of appreciation for the realities of modern healthcare practices among the substance abuse community. In addition, many clinicians doubt that drug abuse prevention works because they treat the illnesses and injuries that result from its failure. As a result, both doctors and prevention activists often are disappointed by the rare collaboration on drug topics.

The expansion of the managed care environment is changing the motivation for doctors to work with prevention. Primary care clinicians have been found to be powerful agents for behavior change in campaigns to reduce tobacco use among adults when given the information they need to intervene effectively. The incentive for reduced tobacco use from the managed care perspective is clear: Less smoking means reduced risk for a wide variety of chronic diseases that will cost the managed care provider a significant amount of money. Mental health interventions have been shown to reduce the stress-related symtoms that account for 30 to 60% of all outpatient visits to primary care physicians (Groth-Marnatt & Edkins, 1996). Similar interest in substance abuse prevention is possible when managed care systems recognize that effective interventions can reduce long-term treatment costs without disrupting the medical provider's routine. As a result, the mid-1990s has seen managed care organizations negotiating cooperative agreements with such traditional substance abuse prevention groups as the local affiliates of the National Council on Alcoholism and Other Drug Dependencies. These alliances benefit both organizations, with the substance abuse prevention groups gaining access to the public at that "golden moment" when people are thinking about health while the managed care system gains credibility as an organization that promotes wellness rather than merely trying to discourage patients from seeking treatment.

PATIENTLY MEASURE SUCCESS

When communities change their physical environment by reducing water pollution or building a transportation network, the public recognizes that these activities take time. For years before a lake is clean enough to swim in or a transit system has enough passengers to make a dent in the rush hour, the community will see these efforts only in terms of the unsightly construction and costs that must be endured.

The same principle is true for drug abuse prevention. Drug abuse takes a long time to develop; the drug problems that we experience today may have their roots in events 30, 50, or even 100 years ago. Getting rid of these problems also takes time and, as a result, requires a permanent structure to monitor progress and make decisions on how to respond.

Americans tend to lack patience. They expect to see a quick return on their investment and are very willing to replace the managers who fail to meet that expectation. On the national level, the state level, and the local level, there is a tendency to frequently move the responsibility for drug abuse prevention from one agency to another without letting much dust settle. And with each change, there are new priorities, new programs, and new initiatives.

Part of the secret to successful drug abuse prevention may be maintaining a stable management team that identifies goals, designs a strategy, and stays together long enough to measure the results. Mark Barnes, drug counsel to the Department of Health and Human Services under President Bush, has argued that such a steadfast, coordinated approach that achieved dramatic progress documented by survey data and other indicators was the core of the national strategy to reduce casual cocaine use during the late 1980s. Critics can question the appropriateness of the goal but no one argues that the Bush Administration failed to meet its targets (Barnes, 1993). The succeeding administration of President Clinton, in contrast, had great difficulty articulating prevention goals in terms of specific reductions of drug abuse, and was seen as less effective in this policy area.

The lesson of the Bush Administration's success in drug abuse prevention applies to prevention efforts at the state and community level. Goals for reduction of targeted substance abuse problems should be clear, measurable, and achievable within a reasonable number of years. The Bush Administration needed to support mechanisms to periodically monitor progress toward the goals and to broadly disseminate reports documenting successful results. The temptation is to garner support by reminding the community how much more work needs to be done, but such grim pronouncements often erode support by suggesting that nothing important has been achieved. In drug abuse prevention, as in any other endeavor, it is better to remind the customers that milestones have been reached rather than point out how much longer the journey will take.

What Doesn't Work
Four Mistakes Preventionists Make

As a general rule, most drug abuse prevention projects that make the effort to conduct a serious evaluation of outcomes can show successful results. Well-documented successes, however, represent only a small fraction of the field. The majority of prevention programs operating during the late 1980s were unwilling or unable to report on a credible evaluation.

Even without enough credible evaluations, it's clear that drug abuse prevention hasn't always delivered success. Every indicator of the total number of drug addicts—as opposed to intermittent drug users—suggests that the people most susceptible to drug dependence continue to fall victim to cocaine and heroin at rates unchanged since the mid-1980s. Communities that faced serious drug problems in the 1980s believe that they continue to face such problems today.

Most disturbingly, despite multimillion dollar investments in school-based prevention, the 1990s witnessed a decline in the percentage of high school seniors who believe that occasional substance abuse is physically harmful. This change in perception was accompanied by an increase in some types of drug use among teenagers; e.g., the percentage of 12th-grade students reporting recent use of LSD doubled between 1991 and 1995 and the percentage who recently used marijuana jumped upwards by 53% (Johnston *et al.*, 1995).

HOW WE KNOW WHAT DOESN'T WORK

Documenting failure can be risky. No evaluator enjoys association with a project that does not reach its goals. Funding sources are uncomfortable providing support to a program that documents a lack of success, especially when competing programs may be willing to hide or even shred disappointing data. When evaluation consultants in the drug abuse field meet informally to "talk shop," a recurrent theme consists of relating how some clients pressure them to portray indifferent outcomes in the best possible light to secure continued funding.

Many advocates for prevention also prefer to explain away evaluation findings that challenge popular or politically comfortable concepts of what should work in prevention. They correctly point out that no researcher can ever be certain that inadequate results are caused by implementation problems rather than a basic design flaw of a prevention program. "If the programs had been adequately funded ... appropriately staffed ... more sensitive to cultural issues, etc.," the advocates suggest, "then these failures would have been successes." Program staff often are accused of being unprepared to carry out prevention activities; program managers sometimes are described as failing to adequately involve community leaders, to mobilize volunteers, or to faithfully replicate a model.[1] According to this reasoning, prevention efforts that produce unimpressive results may really be promising programs that require only tinkering in administration and logistics to succeed.

The flaw in this argument is that community-based drug abuse prevention operates in the real world. It must be a hardy perennial rather than a hothouse blossom. A prevention effort that can be rendered ineffective by routine problems of implementation or administration may have theoretical interest to research but it has limited value to communities trying to cope with real substance abuse problems. At best, well-designed failures illustrate mistakes to be avoided when investing in substance abuse prevention.

Prevention projects that present results of a rigorous evaluation indicating participants generally did not benefit from the intervention or actually experienced poorer outcomes offer important lessons for drug abuse prevention. From them, we learn that some activities and procedures don't work. The following observations on what can go wrong in prevention are based in large part on the comments of managers and evaluators associated with such courageous programs.

THE SELF-ESTEEM TRAP

Self-esteem is the most popular element of a very complex theory of the development of self-concept contributed by Erikson shortly after World War II (Erikson, 1950). Scientists attempted to provide accurate measures for self-esteem, such as the Coopersmith, Piers-Harris, and Rosenberg instruments. The

---

[1] Several of these issues are cited to explain "the lack of overwhelming scientific evidence as to 'what works'" in Abt Associates (1993), *Substance Abuse Prevention: What Works, and Why*, an unpublished paper prepared for the Office of National Drug Control Policy, Executive Office of the President.

creation of these instruments gave rise to the belief that self-esteem is something that can be "fixed" in isolation from other aspects of the personality.

Twenty-five years ago, psychologists studying the causes of addiction conducted clinical interviews with patients in detoxification centers undergoing withdrawal from alcohol or drug dependence. The interviewers discovered a common theme in these interviews, namely, the patients suffered from poor self-esteem. When these scholars attempted to describe an "addictive personality," they often included low self-esteem as a defining characteristic.

Dozens of interventions targeted toward youth today promise that their activities will prevent drug use by improving self-esteem. The creators and managers of everything from sport teams to motivational videotapes claim that their contributions will make children or adolescents "feel good about themselves" and therefore eliminate the need for alcohol or other drugs. In reviewing prevention program outcomes, the single most widely adopted "scientific" instrument is the Rosenberg Self-Esteem Inventory, a diagnostic tool developed during the 1970s for adult assessments.

Most rigorously evaluated programs focusing on self-esteem produce disappointing outcomes (e.g., see Strein, 1988). Youth participants do not consistently improve their scores on the Rosenberg Inventory. In some youth programs, average scores actually decline. In addition, programs that focus on self-esteem rarely if ever demonstrate long-term success in reducing alcohol or drug problems (Gerstein & Green, 1993; Swisher, Doolittle, & Duke, 1994; Schroeder, Laflin, & Weis, 1993).

Many psychologists in the 1990s are uncomfortable with the concept that self-esteem somehow can be separated from the complexity of individual self-image and ego. The creator of the Rosenberg Inventory long argued that monitoring self-esteem does not provide good indications of future behavior. "We will never understand self-esteem," he wrote, "unless we go beyond self-esteem" (Rosenberg, 1979). Even if self-esteem can be analyzed independently from other aspects of personality, researchers generally agree that instruments used by psychologists for measuring self-esteem among adults do not provide meaningful results among young children (see Curry & Johnson, 1990).

In addition to this issue, since the early 1980s, researchers have expressed doubt that a single "addictive personality" exists, in part because it is difficult to imagine a single set of personality characteristics that would serve as a catalyst to addiction to both depressant and stimulant drugs (Lang, 1983). A better explanation for addiction is that certain drugs alter the physical structure of the brain cells of susceptible individuals, so that biological rather than personality characteristics play the critical role in transforming drug use to drug dependence. In addition, some forms of substance abuse, such as LSD use, do not appear to be directly related to the causes of addiction.

A few of the early researchers on common characteristics among patients in detoxification wards now admit that they may have been looking at the wrong end of the chain of drug abuse. The discovery that a nauseated, convulsive alcoholic or addict interviewed in a drunk tank or public asylum has low self-esteem does not reveal anything about the patient's level of self-esteem during first use of alcohol or drugs. When tens of millions of Americans experiment with drugs and a clear majority drink alcoholic beverages, it becomes very difficult to give credence to the claim that abnormally low self-esteem is an important cause of the use of these substances.

A final problem with the self-esteem concept is that adolescents and young children normally show variation in self-esteem, including occasional declines and surges. These variations are not necessarily related to socially approved concerns. For example, adolescents lose self-esteem from romantic rejection, from the acne and voice changes accompanying puberty, and from reluctance to master the complex code of acceptable insults. They may gain self-esteem by hospitalizing a rival or successfully shoplifting. In essence, self-esteem without prosocial values is not necessarily a good thing.

The popularity of self-esteem both as an objective of drug abuse prevention programs and as a measure for success is at least 10 years out of date. If it were possible to isolate and improve self-esteem, and to accurately measure the results, the improvement wouldn't necessarily reduce adolescent substance abuse. A more appropriate goal may be to develop an accurate, positive self-concept that includes realistic expectations for behavior and healthy avoidance of unreasonable risks.

ACTIVITIES FOR THE SAKE OF ACTIVITIES

When prevention program managers gather at conferences and workshops, they often devote their time to exchanging ideas on prevention activities that seemed to work. One preventionist may discuss how children were recruited into a drop-in center by the prospect of self-defense classes. In the same seminar, another site may claim success from promoting a mentoring and literacy improvement effort. A third program may describe a wilderness adventure program that the participants lauded as a highlight of their year.

Some program managers react to such helpful advice by trying to duplicate as many of the successful activities as they can. It is not unusual to find a single prevention effort that attempts to provide education on the consequences of drug use, develop decision-making skills, hold counseling sessions, sponsor mentoring programs, and operate a drop-in center. The same program might also try to improve academic skills, reestablish links to traditional ethnic culture and values, and increase access to recreation and artistic expression. In effect, organizers may assume that if one useful activity is good and two activities are better, then eight activities are better still.

The reality is that the complex prevention programs offering the widest variety of activities may be most likely to fail. There are several possible explanations for the low effectiveness observed among prevention programs with many activities. Running a complex mix of activities may strain the limited management and administrative resources of community-based agencies and coalitions that often accept responsibility for drug abuse prevention. In addition, the attempt to secure resources for activities may divert energy and attention from the basic task of conducting the most effective interventions. For example, an offer of low-cost access to wilderness experience or the opportunity to have a celebrity athlete briefly coach participating youth may be so attractive that it obscures the fundamental question of whether the activity fits into the program. Activities can effectively drive the program rather than vice versa.

Another problem with offering too many choices is that the participants may be so involved in selecting activities—or in competing for inclusion in a favorite pastime with limited enrollment—that the prevention message of the intervention may be lost. For example, one author of this book evaluated a drug abuse prevention effort for approximately 150 inner-city youth that secured 30 slots in a horsemanship program. Children enjoyed the riding lessons, but most program participants were excluded and some resented that the prevention effort did not offer an alternative that they would find equally "fun." The point that all participants were developing skills to cope with the pressures to use drugs vanished in debates about whether children excluded from the horsemanship program would be taken to an amusement park or a wave pool.

The ultimate goal of substance abuse prevention is not to divide the adolescent world between positive, drug-free activities and the activities that youth would engage in without outside intervention. Such a dichotomy potentially reinforces the appearance that there is a world outside of adult supervision in which drugs, sexual activities, risk-taking, and other guilty pleasures are acceptable. The healthier alternative is to promote the concept that drug use should be avoided all of the time, including while engaged in activities that do not earn the approval of the adult world. This suggests that drug abuse prevention should be at least somewhat divorced from the goal of providing youth with supervised recreation and social activities.

In summary, for a variety of reasons, more is not always better when it comes to prevention activities. A few well-chosen activities that mesh with the specific objectives of a prevention effort seem to be more effective than trying to provide many attractive prevention components.

KNOWLEDGE ISN'T ALWAYS POWER

Schools are in the business of fostering knowledge. It therefore is not surprising that many school-based prevention programs, and some programs developed by community agencies and foundations, select prevention "education" efforts that devote considerable time to providing detailed information about drugs and alcohol.

Reviews of prevention programs consistently find that too many targeted at children provide information about how and why people use drugs. Some programs document impressive knowledge gains as suburban youth learn inner-city street names for specific drugs and to describe subjective effects of stimulants and depressants. In most cases, however, such knowledge gains are not associated with significant behavioral change.

Fundamentally, attitudes toward drug use are not necessarily related to the level of information. This should not have been an unexpected finding. Addicts and heavy drug users often are very well informed about the effects and potential consequences of drug use. Experienced consumers of marijuana, for example, can distinguish between the locally grown product and imports from Mexico and South America. Regarding the professions, some doctors and nurses are believed to be frequent abusers of prescription drugs, in part because they assume that their specialized knowledge gives them power over the substance.

On the other side of the use continuum are residents of communities with strong moral and religious prohibitions against drugs, such as fundamentalist Baptists, devout members of the Church of the Latter-Day Saints, and Hasidic Jews. Their relative ignorance of the details of why people use drugs and which drugs are most commonly used does not seem to be a risk factor for drug abuse.

Recognition that helping people to stay well informed about drugs in general does not necessarily result in changing or preventing their drug use behavior resulted in a reaction against drug education by many prevention specialists. This reaction has been helped by evidence from the congressionally mandated National Structured Evaluation of alcohol and drug abuse prevention that the most consistently positive outcomes are reported by programs that do not provide drug "education." In a 1994 address to the National Association of Prevention Professionals and Activists, health educator Richard Clayton flatly argued for the prevention field to abandon drug education as a component of substance abuse prevention.

The reaction against drug education probably should be limited to a reaction against educating the wrong people about the wrong subjects. The Adolescent Alcohol Prevention Trial experiments described in Chapter 5 (Hansen & Graham, 1991) and other studies of drug education curriculum found that use is discouraged among adolescents by providing accurate information on drug use rates among the age group. In effect, many adolescents are dissuaded from engaging in substance abuse by learning that most teenagers do not use drugs, smoke cigarettes, or engage in binge drinking. This knowledge reinforces the image of substance abuse as the characteristic behavior of a "druggie" subculture that most youth do not want to join. Among older youth and adults, substance abuse may be discouraged by accurate discussion of the health and legal consequences of alcohol abuse and drug use.

These types of knowledge gain are very different from the wholesale transmission of facts about which drugs are effective "uppers" and which are "downers" which characterized drug education during the early 1980s. The bottom line appears to be that drug education can be a useful component when it focuses on why people *shouldn't* use drugs rather than attempts to create a well-informed group able to make knowledgeable decisions on substance abuse.

WHEN DRUG ABUSE IS LOGICAL

Many rigorously evaluated programs that could not document favorable outcomes were trying to intervene with very dysfunctional clients. Individuals served by these prevention efforts were often current drug users or had long histories of criminal justice involvement or mental illness. When these programs failed, they typically were attempting to provide only a small dose of intervention among youth who continued to live in desperate conditions. Such programs distribute the equivalent of a Band-Aid to a group whose problems challenge the most comprehensive solutions.

Over 20 years ago, Richard Carney suggested that some drug abuse could be viewed as a rational act:

> Each person chooses those behaviors which at that time, under those circumstances seem to him to have the highest probability of producing need satisfaction (Utility). If this same behavior appears dysfunctional to external observers, it is because they are unable to place themselves into the same decision making position. (Carney, 1974, p. 20)

A heroin addict's explanation for his drug use mirrors Carney's view: "When you're high, you don't notice the rats on your bed or how hungry you are." An individual who never expects to find work, remain healthy, or stay out of jail may rationally decide that the consequences of drug use are outweighed by a few moments of reprieve won from unpleasant reality.

The rationality of drug use under some circumstances cannot justify either legalization or the neglect of prevention among the most hard-to-influence populations: Drug abuse harms society even if it offers temporary benefits to the individual. However, prevention programs must accept that the advantages that individuals obtain from avoiding drug use are not available to some people.

One implication of this observation is that drug abuse prevention conducted in isolation cannot succeed in environments where drug use is a logical and accepted coping mechanism. In most communities, prevention can be effective. In other communities, prevention will succeed only after major improvements in economic and social conditions (e.g., see Dembo, Williams, & Schmeidler, 1994). Absent such change, incentives for drug involvement will often continue to prove more effective than the efforts to keep people away from drugs.

Similarly, we should not assume that every individual has the mental health to react positively toward substance abuse prevention. An individual who suffers from chronic depression is not likely to respond in a predictable manner to a program that attempts to reduce the attractiveness of drug use by improving social interaction skills. A child diagnosed with attention deficit disorder is a poor candidate for a prevention program based on videotapes, puppet shows, or printed materials and lectures. In such cases, the individual may want the benefits of prevention but may be blocked from receiving them by an underlying mental health problem.

This is a very sobering and discouraging point for many preventionists to accept. A workable solution to drug abuse problems, however, depends at least in part on the willingness to admit that preventive interventions are not effective for everyone at risk. Sponsors of a prevention program will do well to adopt a guiding motto of the members of Alcoholics Anonymous: "Our goal is Progress, not Perfection."

Appendix: The National Structured Evaluation on Prevention of Alcohol and Drug Abuse

Most of the prevention programs and projects described in this work were identified and evaluated through the National Structured Evaluation (NSE) study, a project mandated by the U.S. Congress in the Anti-Drug Abuse Act of 1988 (P.L. 100-690). A detailed discussion of the NSE overall findings can be found in the *Third Report to Congress on Alcohol and Other Drug Abuse Prevention: The National Structured Evaluation*, available from the U.S. Department of Health and Human Services. This appendix is included for those who want just a little bit more information on the study.

The NSE study was required to examine virtually every type of activity, other than treatment, that explicitly documented an effort to reduce alcohol and other drug abuse. The responsibility for conducting this evaluation eventually fell to the Center for Substance Abuse Prevention (CSAP), and to Conwal Incorporated, a professional services firm that works closely with CSAP in research and analysis of prevention issues. The directors of the NSE project are the authors of this book.

DATA COLLECTION FOR THE NSE

The decentralization of drug abuse prevention in the United States required 3 years to track down current and recent prevention projects. Prevention efforts operating between 1986—the year of passage of the first comprehensive federal anti-drug abuse legislation—and 1992 were included in the NSE data base. It also included prevention efforts identified through any journal articles published after 1986.

In theory, many programs could qualify under this broad definition of prevention by claiming to indirectly contribute to reducing drug abuse. Participation in traditional afterschool clubs and neighborhood cleanups, for example, fall into this category. In practice, most activities with claims to indirectly reduce drug abuse lack the documentation of effectiveness that would allow inclusion in the NSE.

The other "missing data" in the NSE are the lack of documentation on small prevention efforts funded by local government and private philanthropy. It is unlikely that inclusion of these smaller local and privately funded efforts would have significantly altered the NSE findings. Preliminary results from an extensive national survey of anti-drug abuse initiatives in towns with less than 50,000 population found prevention initiatives that are similar in content to projects funded by direct federal grants. Specifically, locally funded small-town efforts generally focus on D.A.R.E. or a similar school-based curriculum to reach adolescents in school, and adopt a community coalition structure.

The survey also found that small-town prevention efforts conducted without federal support almost never perform systematic evaluation of outcomes (Garofalo & McDermott, 1993). Without outcome data, the inclusion of more small scale local prevention efforts in the NSE would not have helped to assess the effectiveness of these activities.

THE NSE TECHNIQUE FOR ANALYZING EFFECTIVENESS

In addition to data collection, the systematic assessment of approaches to drug abuse prevention posed a large number of methodological challenges. The standard for comparative effectiveness was documentation of specific changes that could reasonably be described as an outcome of the implementation of prevention approaches. To apply this standard, the NSE rated the methodological rigor of evaluations of prevention efforts, so that results of rigorously evaluated prevention efforts could be distinguished from less credible findings. The NSE also had to develop a process to assign an overall rating of effectiveness to prevention efforts that sought to achieve multiple outcomes.

The NSE measured the effectiveness of prevention efforts on the basis of evaluations submitted by the prevention projects themselves. The methodological rigor of these evaluations ranged from barely credible to juried scientific studies, with most evaluations falling somewhere on a continuum between these extremes.

The NSE developed a ten-item assessment for the methodological rigor of prevention program evaluations. The tool allows reviewers to indicate the methodological strengths and weaknesses of each evaluation, and to assign a score ranging from 0 to 5 for overall rigor. Those evaluations scoring 0 were defined as so flawed that no confidence could be placed in the accuracy of the results. A rating of 3 or higher indicated a level of methodological rigor that offered confidence that the direction and general level of outcome reported were accurate. Methodological rigor scores ranging from 1 through 2.5 indicated evaluations whose findings should be used with caution because of lack of adherence to credible evaluation practices. Trial runs of the instrument revealed that four out of five analysts achieved agreement on the rigor rating at least 75% of the time.

At least two senior analysts with advanced training in evaluation methodology independently reviewed each project in the NSE, using the instrument developed for this purpose. Disagreements about the appropriate rating were resolved through consensus. A third senior analyst was always available as a referee if consensus did not emerge; in practice, consensus always was achieved.

The NSE staff considered limiting the rating process to prevention efforts that used rigorous evaluation to measure effects on the rates of drug use. Unfortunately, drug abuse prevention does not provide clean, comparable measures of behavior change. Behavior change is measured by indicators selected by each prevention effort—sometimes with guidance from competent, professional evaluators and sometimes without such guidance. Three examples illustrate how this makes life difficult for evaluation:

■ In one program, the data suggest that the prevention effort had an impact on marijuana use—but produced no significant change on other drug use. Should this effort be viewed as a qualified success, or as a failure?
■ The data in another program could reflect either reduced drug use in the community or reduced community interest in enforcement of laws on drug possession. How should such data be viewed in comparative perspective?
■ A third program concentrated on beer and wine and measured change in frequency and quantity of consumption. How should these results be compared with those of programs that measure complete abstinence?

These three cases all measure behavior changes immediately on completion of the prevention program. Other evaluations track behavior change from 3 months to 5 years after participation in a prevention effort. Such differences in timing of follow-up make comparisons even more difficult.

Broadening the scope of evaluation to include changes in knowledge about drugs and attitudes toward drugs offered benefits to the comparability of projects in the NSE. Knowledge and attitude changes tend to be measured according to standard criteria, such as pretest/posttest changes on questionnaire responses. Even these measurements, however, can vary among programs.

Many prevention projects targeting young children do not attempt to measure drug use or drug-related attitudes and knowledge. These projects often address potential precursors of future drug problems, including academic failure, conduct issues, and social and emotional adjustment problems. Using such risk and protective factors as a gauge of performance is a reasonable measure of success given the very low rates of alcohol and drug use among young children.

Finally, many prevention efforts do not seek to attain only one objective; a school-based prevention effort may simultaneously try to prevent initiation of marijuana use, reduce frequency of alcohol consumption, increase knowledge about the consequences of drug use, improve school grades, and increase the rates of referral of families to social service intervention.

Instead of struggling to fit all programs into a common measure for all types of prevention outcomes, the NSE measured effectiveness independently among three categories of change:

- *Change in behavior directly related to alcohol and other drug use.* This category includes changes in the frequency and quantity of consumption, in the frequency of especially risky use (e.g., drinking before driving, smoking during pregnancy), and in rates of initiation of alcohol, tobacco, and other drug use.
- *Change in knowledge and attitudes directly related to alcohol and other drugs.* This category includes changes in survey responses on attitudes and expectations regarding drug use, as well as changes in scores on instruments that measure knowledge of the nature and consequences of alcohol and other drug use.
- *Change in risk and protective factors.* This category includes measurable changes in all areas that may affect future use of alcohol and other drugs, including academic and work-related performance, cultural values, involvement in crime, social skills, mental and physical health, quality of family life and support.

The NSE discovered that experienced prevention researchers and evaluators, operating independently, could agree about the apparent effectiveness for these categories of change. The NSE overcame the problems of chaotic outcomes to present broad comparisons of relative effectiveness among programs in the field.

The NSE opted to employ a modified Q-sort procedure: basically the same technique that a teacher uses to grade test papers. Just as a teacher uses grades ranging from A through F, the raters also assigned projects to five categories of effectiveness:

5	Significant effectiveness
4	Moderate effectiveness
3	Limited effectiveness, but generally positive
2	No net impact
1	Negative impact

One concern raised about a Q-sort approach was that expert raters might disagree about what constitutes effectiveness. To rule out this possibility, the NSE asked nine highly qualified raters working in seven cities to independently evaluate 137 randomly selected projects. The results of the independent rating efforts were remarkably similar. The nine raters scored better than 0.750 on an index of intercoder agreement for drug behavior outcomes, knowledge and attitude outcomes, and risk/protective factor outcomes. The agreement on appropriate "grades" among nine independent judges was up to 9 times better than chance for the three outcome categories.

The pilot test then was duplicated with seven additional senior analysts with expertise in prevention. Similar results were obtained: The second panel of judges achieved better than 0.80 agreement with the first panel on the ratings for all alcohol and drug abuse prevention projects.

THE SEVEN DRUG ABUSE PREVENTION APPROACHES

A statistical technique known as cluster analysis was used to divide prevention programs into groups based on similarities in the mix of activities. This procedure identified a stable set of seven distinct approaches to drug abuse prevention:

- *Positive Decision-making Approach* Provided *only* personal skills development and didactic drug education ("personal skills" refer to mental health, and social skills that apply to a wide variety of situations including generic decision-making, assertiveness, coping, and interpersonal skills).
- *Safety/Health Skills Approach* Provided personal skills development, didactic drug *and* safety education.
- *Psychosocial Skills Approach* Provided personal skills development *and/or* task-oriented skill training *without* drug education ("task-ori-

ented skills training" refers to acquisition of a skill or ability used to perform a specific task. Such skills include parenting skills, academic skills, and job-seeking skills).

■ *Counseling Intensive Approach* Provided interpersonal counseling and/or family intervention, *and* education on drug use effects. "interpersonal counseling," as used in the NSE, does not include either addiction treatment or mentoring activities; these were placed in separate activity categories.

■ *Case Management Approach* Provided case management, interpersonal counseling, *and* task-oriented skills training.

■ *Multidirectional Approach* Provided many activities including, at a minimum, drug education, both personal skills and task-oriented skills training, and access to drug-free cultural and recreational activities.

■ *Environmental Change Approach* Activities that change the community environment without directly intervening with individuals at risk of alcohol or other drug-related problems.

A summary of this typology appears in Table A.1. Table A.2 describes the principal findings for each of the seven approaches in terms of the populations and communities served in the identified examples.

Highlights of findings about the approaches include

■ The limited activity mix defined as the *Positive Decision-making* approach dominated prevention efforts for preadolescent children.

■ The activity mix of the *Psychosocial Skills* approach typically was administered by nonprofit agencies. Surprisingly few examples of this skill-building approach were directed at young children.

■ A relatively large number of programs using the *Counseling Intensive* approach were operated by government agencies. Over one-third of prevention efforts directed at Spanish-speaking communities use this approach.

■ Despite a similar activity mix, the *Case Management* approach differed from the *Counseling Intensive* approach in several significant characteristics, including a tendency toward much longer duration of client participation and involvement of healthcare and/or addiction professionals as primary facilitators. Because the *Case Management* approach included efforts under the Pregnant/Postpartum Women and Infants prevention grants, it offered most of the identified cases of gender-specific prevention in the NSE.

■ The *Environmental Change* approach was widely used throughout the United States. School-administered prevention efforts, however, were least likely to engage in environmental change activities.

Table A.1. Activity Characteristics of the Seven Approaches to AOD Abuse
Prevention

Approach	Defining activity mix	Other activities often included
Positive decision-making (147 cases)	Personal skills development and/or education on effects of drug use, with no other activities	None
Safety/health skills (15 cases)	Personal skills development, education on effects of drug use, and safety education	General health and wellness education and/ or task-oriented skills training
Psychosocial skills (68 cases)	Personal skills development, task-oriented skill training, with no drug education	Drug-free cultural or recreational activities *or* a wilderness challenge experience
Counseling intensive (67 cases)	Interpersonal and/or family counseling, and education on the effects of drug use	Personal skills development and task-oriented skills training
Case management (48 cases)	Case management, interpersonal counseling, and task-oriented skills training	Treatment for addiction, "drug education," and referral to other service providers
Multidirectional (81 cases)	At least six types of activities, including education on effects of drug use, personal and task-oriented skills training, and drug-free recreational and cultural activities	Interpersonal counseling, health education, and cultural regrounding for ethnic minorities
Environmental change (209 cases)	Activities to change the community environment such as training professionals who work with children, forming prevention coalitions, and revising laws or enforcement patterns to restrict effective access to alcohol, tobacco, and other drugs	

As expected, no single approach emerged as consistently superior in effectiveness across all types of outcome and all populations. Instead, the NSE data suggest a complex pattern of relative strengths and weaknesses, some of which may be specific to individual age groups

- Identified examples of the *Positive Decision-making* approach included some prevention efforts that were clearly outstanding both in methodological rigor and in effectiveness. Overall, implementation of the approach tended to yield best results in terms of change in knowledge and attitudes for adolescent populations and in reducing drug problems among adult populations. Among younger participants, *Positive Decision-making* programs typically were rated lower in effectiveness than other approaches.

Table A.2. Client and Host Community Characteristics of the Seven Approaches to AOD Abuse Prevention

Approach	Population characteristics	Host communities
Positive decision-making	Defines most prevention directed specifically at preadolescent children. Less likely to be used among older youth and adults	Smaller cities and towns (urban places with less than 250,000 population) were most likely to host this approach
Safety/health skills	Majority served only adolescent participants	More common among relatively high-income communities
Psychosocial skills	Nearly 30% of identified cases served older teens and/or adult clients. Relatively infrequently applied to preadolescent children	Most popular in rural jurisdictions. Suburban communities least likely to host approach
Counseling intensive	Most examples served older youth and adults. Among minority ethnic groups, most widely-reported among Hispanic-American programs	Most examples were hosted in large cities (i.e., over 250,000 population)
Case management	Two-thirds of cases served adult participants. Typical of the Pregnant and postpartum Women and Infants programs (see Chapter 2)	Nearly all cases were found either within a central city or in a close-in suburb
Multidirectional	Nearly half served minority ethnic schoolchildren: 28% had exclusively African-American clients	60% of all identified cases were hosted in neighborhoods of large cities
Environmental change	Most examples not directed at specific demographic subgroup	Widely distributed among community types but least typical of large cities

■ Identified examples of prevention efforts adopting the *Psychosocial Skills* approach generally achieved positive change in terms of both problem behaviors and long-term risk and protective factors. The approach appeared less successful in affecting factual knowledge and conscious attitudes. Although few examples of the approach were rated as truly outstanding in effectiveness, *Psychosocial Skills* programs achieved good results for a wide variety of populations and settings, including preadolescent children.

■ Identified examples of the *Counseling Intensive* approach generally received low ratings for effectiveness. However, 70% of the examples of the approach designed to affect long-term risk and protective factors among adolescents at risk were rated effective.

■ The *Case Management* approach included several rigorously evaluated programs that clearly document behavior change. It achieved a high mean effectiveness rating for reducing drug use problem behavior and for influencing risk/protective factors among adults and among older adolescents.

The *Multidirectional* approach included a few cases of effective outcomes among adolescents. However, most uses of the approach did not demonstrate effective performance for any type of outcome among any population.

Examples of the *Environmental Change* approach included some of the most effective programs and had the most consistent record of effectiveness across all types of outcomes.

Additional findings from the NSE were incorporated in the *Third Report to Congress on Alcohol and Other Drug Abuse Prevention of the Secretary of Health and Human Services*, released in September, 1995.

References

Abt Associates. (1993). *Substance abuse prevention: What works, and why*. An unpublished paper prepared for the Office of National Drug Control Policy, Executive Office of the President.

Allen, G. A. (1991). *Annual report of The Family Circles Program*. Unpublished report submitted to the Center for Substance Abuse Prevention, Rockville, MD.

Andrews, J. A., Hops, H., Ary, D. V., Tildesley, E., & Harris, J. (1993). Parental influences on early adolescent substance use: Specific and non-specific effects. *Journal of Early Adolescence, 13*, 285–310.

Atkinson, R. M., Tolson, R. L., & Turner, J. A. (1990). Late versus early onset problem drinking in older men. *Alcohol Clinical and Experimental Research, 14*, 574–579.

Baer, J. S., Kivlahan, D. R., Fromme, K., & Marlatt, G. A. (1991). Secondary prevention of alcohol abuse with college student populations: A skills-training approach. In N. Heather, W. Miller, & J. Greeley (Eds.), *Self-control and the addictive behaviors* (pp. 338–354). Botany, Australia: Maxwell Macmillan Publishing Australia.

Barnes, M. (1993). Drug policy under the Bush administration: Assessing its strengths and weaknesses. Unpublished presentation to the 121st annual meeting of the American Public Health Association, October 26, San Francisco, CA.

Bonthius, D. J., & West, J. R. (1989). Blood alcohol concentration and microencephaly. *Journal of Alcohol Clinical and Experimental Research, 14*, 107–118.

Botvin, G. S., Baker, E., Dusenbury, L., Botvin, E. M., & Diaz, T. (1995). Long-term follow-up results of a randomized drug abuse prevention trial in a white middle-class population. *Journal of the American Medical Association, 273*, 1106–1112.

Brook, J. S., Whiteman, M., Gordon, A. S., & Brook, D. W. (1990). The role of older brothers in younger brothers' drug use view in the context of parent and peer influences. *Journal of Genetic Psychology, 15*, 59–75.

Caetano, R., & Medina-Mora, M. E. (1990). Reasons and attitudes toward drinking and abstaining: Comparison of Mexicans and Mexican-Americans. *Epidemiologic trends in drug use: Community Epidemiology Work Group proceedings, June 1990* (pp. 173–191). Rockville, MD: National Institute on Drug Abuse.

Camilli, G., & Brennan, T. (1984). *An evaluation of the "Alcohol, Drugs, Driving and You" curriculum project*. Unpublished manuscript available from The Prevention Center, Charlotte, NC.

Caplan, M., Weissberg, R. P., Grober, J. S., Sivo, P. J., Grady, K., & Jacoby, C. (1992). Social competence promotion with inner-city and suburban young adolescents: Effects on social adjustment and alcohol use. *Journal of Consulting and Clinical Psychology, 60*, 56–63.

Carney, R. E. (1974). A risk-taking, valuing approach to evalution of programs to modify problem behaviors. Unpublished paper disseminated by Educators Assistance Institute, Santa Monica, CA.

Casement, M. R. (1987). Alcohol and cocaine. *Alcohol Health & Research World, 11*, 18–19.

Center for Substance Abuse Prevention. (1995). *National evaluation of the Community Partnership Demonstration Program Phase II, fourth annual report.* Unpublished report submitted to the Office for Scientific Analysis, Center for Substance Abuse Prevention.

Chaiken, M. R. (1990). Evaluation of Girls Clubs of America's Friendly PEERsuasion program. In R. R. Watson (Ed.), *Drug and alcohol abuse prevention* (pp. 95–132). Clifton, NJ: Humana Press.

Curry, N. E., & Johnson, C. N. (1990). *Beyond self-esteem: Developing a genuine sense of human value.* Washington, DC: National Association for the Education of Young Children.

DeJong. W. (1987). A short term evaluation of Project DARE (Drug Abuse Resistance Education): Preliminary indications of effectiveness, *Journal of Drug Education,* 17(4), 279–294.

Dembo, R., Williams, A., & Schmeidler, J. (1994). Psychosocial, alcohol/ other drug use, and delinquency differences between urban black and white male high risk youth. *International Journal of the Addictions, 29,* 461–483.

Dinkmeyer, D. & McKay, G. (1976). *Systematic training for effective parenting.* Circle Pines, MN: American Guidance Service.

Dishion, T. J., & Andrews, D. W. (1995). Preventing escalation in problem behaviors with high-risk young adolescents. *Journal of Clinical and Consulting Psychology, 63,* 538–548.

DuBose, D. E., Scaglione, R. M., Jordan, L. M., Vaughn, D. A., Fournier, R., & Royal, J. L. C. (1992). *Drug prevention and reduction services to runaway and homeless youth.* New Haven: Youth Continuum, Inc.

Dukes, R. L. (1989). *An evaluation of the 1989 DARE Program in Colorado.* Unpublished paper released by the Center for Social Science Research, University of Colorado, Colorado Springs.

Eggert, L. L., & Herting, J. R. (1991). Preventing teenage drug abuse: Exploratory effects of network social support. *Youth and Society, 22,* 482–524.

Eggert, L. L., Seyl, C. D., & Nicholas, L. J. (1990). Effects of a school-based prevention program for potential high school dropouts and drug abusers. *International Journal of the Addictions, 25,* 773–801.

Eggert, L. L., Thompson, E. A., Herting, J. A., Nicholas, L. J., & Dicker, B. G. (1994). Preventing adolescent drug abuse and high school dropout through an intensive school-based social network development program. *American Journal of Health Promotion, 8(3),* 202–215.

Elkin, D., & Bowen, R. (1979). Imaginary audience behavior in children and adolescents. *Developmental Psychology, 15,* 38–44.

Ellickson, P. L., & Bell, R. M. (1990). Drug prevention in junior high: A multi-site longitudinal test. *Science, 247,* 1299–1305.

Ellickson, P. L., Bell, R. M., & Harrison, E. R. (1993). Changing adolescent propensities to use drugs: Results from Project ALERT. *Health Education Quarterly, 20,* 227–242.

Erikson, E. (1950). *Childhood and society.* New York: Norton.

Errecart, M. T., Walberg, H. J., Ross, J. G., Gold, R. S., Fiedler, J. L., & Kolbe, L. J. (1991). Effectiveness of Teenage Health Teaching Modules. *Journal of School Health, 61,* 26–30.

Faulk, R., & Delaney, B. (1993). *Everyday Theater, Inc. Progress report for March to August, 1993.* Unpublished report submitted to the Center for Substance Abuse Prevention, Rockville, MD.

Fell, J. C. (1988). *The need for a multidisciplinary approach to reduce drinking, driving, and injury.* Unpublished paper presented to the National Trauma Symposium, Baltimore.

Fleming, L., & Davis, T. (1987). *Final report of the "Alcohol, Drugs, Driving, and You" 1986 National Demonstration Program.* Unpublished manuscript available from The Prevention Center, Charlotte, NC.

Fraiberg, S. H. (1959). *The magic years.* New York: Scribner's.

Garofalo, J., & McDermott, J. (1993). *Drugs in small cities and towns: A national study of perceptions of the problem and programmatic solutions.* Unpublished presentation to the 121st annual meeting of the American Public Health Association, October 27, San Francisco, CA.

Gerstein, D. R., & Green, L. W. (1993). *Preventing drug abuse: What do we know?* Washington, DC: National Research Council.

Glider, P., Kressler, H., & McGrew, G. (1991). *Prevention/early intervention through peer support retreats.* Unpublished manuscript distributed by Amity, Inc., Tucson, AZ.

Golub, A., & Johnson, B. D. (1994). A recent decline in cocaine use among youthful arrestees in Manhatten. *American Journal of Public Health, 84,* 1250–1254.

Groth-Marnat, G., & Edkins, G. (1996). Professional psychologists in general health care settings: A review of the financial efficacy of direct treatment interventions. *Professional Psychology: Research and Practice, 27*(2), 161–174.

Hansen, W. B., & Graham, J. W. (1991). Preventing alcohol, marijuana, and cigarette use among adolescents. *Preventive Medicine, 20,* 414–430.

Harrington, C. R., Putnam, S. L., Waters, W. J., & Colt, A. M. (1989). The community gatekeeper training model for reducing alcohol abuse and alcohol-related injury. *Rhode Island Medical Journal, 72,* 459–463.

Hawkins, J. D., Catalano, R. F., & Miller, J. Y. (1992). Risk and protective factors for alcohol and other drug problems. *Psychological Bulletin, 112,* 64–105.

Hawkins, J. D., Catalano, R. F., Morrison, D. M., O'Donnell, J., Abbott, R. D., & Day, L. E. (1992). The Seattle Social Development Project: Effects of the first four years on protective factors and problem behaviors. In J. McCord and R. E. Tremblay (Eds.), *Preventing antisocial behavior: Interventions from birth to adolescence* (pp. 139–161). New York: Guilford Press.

Hawkins, J. D., von Cleve, E., & Catalano, R. F. (1991). Reducing early childhood aggression: Results of a primary prevention program. *Journal of the American Academy of Child and Adolescent Psychology, 3,* 208–217.

Hecht, M. L., Corman, S. R., & Miller-Rassulo, M. (1993). An evaluation of the Drug Resistance Project. *Health Communications, 5,* 75–88.

Holder, H. D., Janes, K., Mosher, J., Saltz, R. F., Spurr, S., & Wagenaar, A. C. (1993). Alcoholic beverage server liability and the reduction of alcohol-involved problems. *Journal of Studies on Alcohol, 54,* 23–36.

Hughes, J. N., & Cavell, T. A. (1995). *Integrative home–school intervention for aggressive children.* Unpublished paper presented to the 103rd annual meeting of American Psychological Association, New York City.

Huhn, R. P., & Zimpfer, D. G. (1989). Effects of a parent education program on parents and their preadolescent children. *Journal of Community Psychology, 17,* 311–318.

Johnston, L. D., O'Malley, P. M., & Bachman, J. G. (1995). *The Monitoring the Future Study, 1995.* Rockville, MD: U. S. Department of Health and Human Services.

Join Together. (1996). Leading from the ground up—The Third National Survey of the Community Movement Against Substance Abuse. Boston: Author.

Kim, S., McLeod, J. H., & Shantzis, C. (1990). A short-term outcome evaluation of the "I'm Special" drug abuse prevention program. *Journal of Drug Education, 20,* 127–138.

Klitzner, M., Bamberger, E., & Gruenewald, P. J. (1990) The assessment of parent-led prevention programs: A national descriptive study. *Journal of Drug Education, 20,* 111–125.

Klitzner, M., Gruenewald, P. J., & Bamberger, E. (1990) The assessment of parent-led prevention programs: A preliminary assessment of impact. *Journal of Drug Education, 20,* 77–94.

Koop, C. E. (1995). Editorial: A personal role in health care reform. *American Journal of Public Health, 85,* 759–760.

Kumpfer, K. L. (1992). *Strengthening America's families*. Rockville, MD: Office of Juvenile Justice and Delinquency Prevention, Juvenile Justice Resource Clearinghouse.

Lang, A. R. (1983). Addictive personality: A viable construct? In P. K. Levinson, D. R. Gerstein, & D. R. Maloff (Eds.), *Commonalities in substance abuse and habitual behavior* (pp. 157–236). Boston: Heath.

LoSciuto, L., & Ausetts, M. A. (1988). Evaluation of a drug abuse prevention program: A field experiment. *Addictive Behaviors, 13*, 337–351.

MacKinnon, D. P., Johnson, C. A., Pentz, M. A., Dwyer, J. H., Hansen, W. B., Flay, B. R., & Wang, E. Y. (1991). Mediating mechanisms in a school-based drug prevention program: First year effects. *Health Psychology, 10*, 164–172.

Macro International. (1993). *Final report—CSAP PPWI Demonstration Program findings*. Unpublished report submitted to the Center for Substance Abuse Prevention, Rockville, MD.

May, P. A., & Hymbaugh, K. J. (1983). A pilot project on fetal alcohol syndrome among American Indians. *Alcohol Health & Research World, 7*, 3–9.

May, P. A., & Hymbaugh, K. J. (1989). A macro-level fetal alcohol syndrome prevention program for Native Americans and Alaska Natives. *Journal of Studies on Alcohol, 50*, 508–518.

McKnight, A. J. (1991). Factors influencing the effectiveness of server intervention education. *Journal of Studies on Alcohol, 52*, 389–398.

Midanik, L. T., & Clark, W. B. (1994). The demographic distribution of U. S. drinking patterns in 1990. *American Journal of Public Health, 84*, 1218–1222.

Minnis, J. (1990). Alcohol and aging: A review of the literature. *The Southwestern, 7*, 7–32.

Moody, K. A., & Eggert, L. L. (1992). Exploratory effects of a social support intervention for high-risk youth. Paper prepared for publication.

Morehouse, E. R., Tobler, N., & Kleinman, P. H. (1995). *Comprehensive student assistance in residential setting*. Unpublished final research report submitted to the Center for Substance Abuse Prevention, Rockville, MD.

Morse, B. J., & Elliott, D. S. (1992). Effects of ignition interlock devices on DUI recidivism. *Crime & Delinquency, 38*, 131–157.

National Institute on Alcohol Abuse and Alcoholism. (1995). *The physicians' guide to helping patients with alcohol problems* (NIH Publication No. 95–3769). Bethesda, MD: National Institutes of Health.

National Institute on Drug Abuse. (1996). *Proceedings of the research meeting on drug abuse prevention through family interventions*, January 25–26, 1996, Gaithersburg, MD.

Pentz, M. A., MacKinnon, D. P., Dwyer, J. P., Wang, E. Y., Hansen, W. B., Flay, B. R., & Johnson, C. A. (1989a). Longitudinal effects of the Midwest Prevention Project on regular and experimental smoking in adolescents. *Preventive Medicine, 18*, 304–321.

Pentz, M. A., MacKinnon, D. P., Dwyer, J. P., Wang, E. Y., Hansen, W. B., Flay, B. R., & Johnson, C. A. (1989b). A multi-community trial for primary prevention of adolescent drug abuse. *Journal of the American Medical Association, 261*, 3259–3267.

Pentz, M. A., Johnson, A., Hansen, W., Flay, B., Dwyer, J., & MacKinnon, D. P. (1991). *Effects of community-based drug abuse prevention for adolescents*. Presented to the annual meeting of the American Public Health Association, Atlanta.

Perkins, H. W. (1994). *Misperceptions of alcohol and other drug norms in the collegiate environment*. Presented to the annual meeting of the American Public Health Association, Washington, DC.

Piaget J. (1950). *The psychology of intelligence*. London: Routledge & Kegan Paul.

Prinz, R. J., & Miller, G. E. (1994). Family-based treatment for childhood antisocial behavior. *Journal of Consulting and Clinical Psychology, 62*, 645–650.

Rhode Island Department of Health (1989). *Final report of the Rhode Island Community Alcohol Abuse and Injury Prevention Project*. Unpublished paper submitted to the Centers for Disease

Control in Atlanta, and to the National Institute on Alcohol Abuse and Alcoholism in Bethesda, Maryland, in fulfillment of research grants.

Ringwalt, C., Ennett, S. T., & Holt, K. D. (1991). *An outcome evaluation of Project DARE.* Unpublished paper released by the Center for Social Research and Policy Analysis, Research Triangle Institute, Research Triangle Park, NC 27709–2194.

Ringwalt, C., Curtis, T. R., & Rosenbaum, D. (1990). *A first-year evaluation of D. A. R. E. in Illinois.* Unpublished study prepared for the Illinois State Police.

Rogers, D. E., & Ginzberg, E., (Eds.). (1992). *Adolescents at risk: Medical and social perspectives.* New Haven: Westview Press.

Rosenberg, M. (1979). *Conceiving the self.* New York: Basic Books.

Russ, N. W., & Geller, E. S. (1987). Training bar personnel to prevent drunken driving: A field evaluation. *American Journal of Public Health, 77,* 952–954.

Saltz, R. F. (1987). The roles of bars and restaurants in preventing alcohol-impaired driving. *Evaluation and Health Professions, 10,* 5–27.

Saltz, R. F. (1989). Research needs and opportunities in server intervention programs. *Health Education, 16,* 429–438.

Schinke, S. P., Cole, K. C., & Orlandi, M. A. (1991). *The effects of Boys and Girls Clubs on alcohol and other drug use and related problems in public housing.* Unpublished research report submitted to the Center for Substance Abuse Prevention, Rockville, MD.

Schroeder, D. S., Laflin, M. T., & Weis, D. L. (1993). Is there a relationship between self-esteem and drug use? Methodological and statistical limitations of the research. *Journal of Drug Issues, 23,* 645–655.

Shope, J. T., Copeland, L. A., Maharg, R., Dielman, T. E., & Butchart, A. T. (1993). Assessment of adolescent refusal skills in an alcohol misuse prevention study. *Health Education Quarterly, 20,* 373–390.

Stout, R. L., Rose, J. S., Speare, M. C., Buka, S. L., Laforge, R. G., Campbell, M. K., & Waters, W. J. (1992). *Sustaining interventions in communities.* Unpublished paper submitted to the 2nd International Symposium on Experiences With Community Action Projects for Prevention of Alcohol and Other Drug Problems.

Strein, N. (1988). Classroom-based elementary school affective education programs: A critical review. *Psychology in the Schools, 25,* 288–296.

Substance Abuse and Mental Health Services Administration (SAMHSA), Office of Applied Studies. (1995). *National household survey on drug abuse: Population estimates 1994* (DHHS Publication No. (SMA) 95-3063). Rockville, MD: U.S. Department of Health and Human Services, Public Health Service.

Swisher, J. D., Doolittle, R. H., & Duke, L. (1994). *School based prevention impacts on substances and violence.* Paper presented to the 122nd annual meeting of the American Public Health Association, Washington, DC.

Szapocznik, J., Santisteban, A., Rio, A., Perez-Vidal, A., Santisteban, D., & Kurtines, W. M. (1989). Family Effectiveness Training: An intervention to prevent drug abuse and problem behaviors in Hispanic adolescents. *Hispanic Journal of Behavioral Sciences, 11,* 4–27.

Tobler, N., Kleinman, P., Morehouse, E., & Barkley, D. (1991). *Comparison of substance use by high risk adolescents in residential settings with the National H. S. Senior Survey.* Unpublished evaluation study submitted to the Center for Substance Abuse Prevention, Rockville, MD.

Weinberg, N. Z., Dielman, T. E., Mandell, W., & Shope, J. T. (1994). Parental drinking and gender factors in prediction of early adolescent alcohol use. *International Journal of the Addictions, 29,* 89–104.

Williams, G. D., & DeBakey, S. F. (1992). Changes in level of alcohol consumption. *British Journal of Addiction, 87,* 643–648.

Williams, G. D., Stinson, E. S., Brooks, S. D., Clem, D., & Noble, J. (1991). *Apparent per capita alcohol consumption: National, state, and regional trends, 1977–1989* (NIAAA Surveillance Report No. 20). Washington, DC: U. S. Government Printing Office.

Wodarski, J. S. (1987). Teaching adolescents about alcohol and driving: A two-year follow-up. *Journal of Drug Education, 17,* 327–344.

Wodarski, L. A., Adelson, C. L., Todd, M. T., & Wodarski, J. S. (1980). Teaching nutrition by Teams–Games–Tournaments. *Journal of Nutrition Education, 12,* 61–65.

Wolfson, M., Forster, J. L., Finnegan, J. R., Wagenaar, A. C., Williams, C. L., Perry, C. L., & Anstine, P. (1992). *Opinions of community leaders, alcohol merchants, parents, and students about adolescent alcohol use and problems.* Presented at the 120th annual meeting of the American Public Health Association, Washington, DC.

Worden, J. K., Flynn, B. S., Merrill, D. G., Waller, J. A., & Haugh, L. D. (1989). Preventing alcohol-impaired driving through community self-regulation training. *American Journal of Public Health, 79,* 287–290.

Index

Transportation of clients (*cont.*)
  in Project Network, 23
  in Strengthening Black Families, 34

Values content of mental health promotion, 44–
  45
Violence: *see* Antisocial behavior

Volunteers
  compared to mental health professionals, 40–41
  in Midwest Prevention Program, 151
  in New Start, 20
  profiled, 30

Winter Comforts, 123–124